Occupational Health

Edited by Sheila Pantry OBE

Sheila Pantry Associates
Sheffield
UK

CHAPMAN & HALL

London · Glasgow · Weinheim · New York · Tokyo · Melbourne · Madras

Published by Chapman & Hall, 2–6 Boundary Row, London SE1 8HN, UK

Chapman & Hall, 2–6 Boundary Row, London SE1 8HN, UK

Blackie Academic & Professional, Wester Cleddens Road, Bishopbriggs, Glasgow G64 2NZ, UK

Chapman & Hall GmbH, Pappelallee 3, 69469 Weinheim, Germany

Chapman & Hall USA, 115 Fifth Avenue, New York NY 10003, USA

Chapman & Hall Japan, ITP-Japan, Kyowa Building, 3F, 2-2-1 Hirakawacho, Chiyoda-ku, Tokyo 102, Japan

Chapman & Hall Australia, Thomas Nelson Australia, 102 Dodds Street, South Melbourne, Victoria 3205, Australia

Chapman & Hall India, R. Seshadri, 32 Second Main Road, CIT East, Madras 600 035, India

Distributed in the USA and Canada by Singular Publishing Group Inc., 4284 41st Street, San Diego, California 92105

First edition 1995

© 1995 Sheila Pantry

Typeset in Palatino 10/12 pt by Best-set Typesetter Ltd, Hong Kong
Printed in Great Britain by T.J. Press (Padstow) Ltd.

ISBN 0 412 60410 8   1 56593 415 6 (USA)

A catalogue record for this book is available from the British Library

Library of Congress Catalog Card Number: 94-74706

Contents

Contributors

Jukka Takala
International Labour Office
Occupational Safety and Health
    International Information
    Centre, CIS
Geneva
Switzerland

Paul Lloyd
Consultant in Occupational
    Health
22 Queensway
Penwortham
Preston
UK

Terry ap Hywel
8 Pembroke Court
Caerphilly
UK

Jean Raper
Principal Occupational Health
    Nurse
Sheffield City Council
Sheffield
UK

Kit Artus
Artus Associates
Reading
UK

Steve Fairhurst
Health and Safety Executive
Bootle
UK

Ted Megaw
Industrial Ergonomics Group
School of Manufacturing and
    Mechanical Engineering
The University of Birmingham
Birmingham
UK

Stephen Bailey
Flexpro
1 Chanctonbury View
Henfield
UK

Matthew C. Cullen
Occupational Health Nurse
    Consultant
21 Westwood Road
Manchester
UK

Indira Ashton
Divisional Safety Manager
AWE
Aldermaston
UK

Ian Wright
SmithKline Beecham
   Pharmaceutical
Worthing
UK

James Garvey
Manchester Metropolitan
   University
Elizabeth Gaskell Campus
Manchester
UK

Sheila Pantry OBE
Sheila Pantry Associates
Sheffield
UK

Foreword

As befits her vocation as an information services consultant, Sheila Pantry has brought together a remarkable compendium of information about occupational health. Probably no one would read this collection of authoritative articles from end to end; but nowhere else would a reader be able to find a 'way in' to all the relevant issues, and her own excellent summary of the main sources of information will carry the enquirer further – as far as she or he can go.

The subject of occupational health is developing quickly. We now realize that far more people meet a premature death each year due to their health having been harmed at work than are killed in accidents either at work or due to work activity.

The evidence is also that more people are obliged to give up work prematurely for health reasons than because they have met with an accident. We realize as well that whereas the trend for accidents is clearly favourable, we simply do not know what the trend for health effects is. This book is a useful departure point for the further knowledge that we all need to gain.

J. D. Rimington CB
Director General
Health and Safety Executive

Glossary

FLP	Functional Limits Programme
FWS	Fieldwork Supervisor
GNP	Gross National Product
GP	General Practitioner
HCM	Health Career Model
HPV	High Production Volume
HSC	Health and Safety Commission
HSE	Health and Safety Executive
HSFAR	Health and Safety (First Aid) Regulations
ILO/CIS	International Labour Office Health and Safety Centre (in Geneva, Switzerland; CIS are the French initials)
IOSH	Institution of Occupational Safety and Health
IPCS	International Programme on Chemical Safety
ICRP	International Council for Radiological Protection
ILO	International Labour Office (in Geneva)
JAMA	Journal of the American Medical Association
LOAEL	Lowest Observed Adverse Effect Level
MEE	Methods of Enquiry and Evaluation
MELs	Maximum Exposure Limits
MMU	Manchester Metropolitan University
NCVQ	National Council for Vocational Qualifications
NHP	Nottingham Health Programme
NIOSH	National Institute of Occupational Safety and Health (in USA)
NOAEL	No Observed Adverse Effect Level
NONS	Notification of New Substances Regulations
NVQ	National Vocational Qualification
OECD	Organization for Economic Co-operation and Development (Paris, France)
OELs	Occupational Exposure Limits
OESs	Occupational Exposure Standards
OH	Occupational Health
OHN	Occupational Health Nurse
OHNC	Occupational Health Nursing Certificate
OHSLB	Occupational Health and Safety Lead Body
OHNTAG	Occupational Health Nurse Training Advisory Group
OPCS	Office of Population Censuses and Surveys
OSHA	Occupational Safety and Health Administration (in USA)
OSHIG	Occupational Safety and Health Information Group
OWAS	Ovako Working Posture Analysis System
PACT	Placement Assessment and Counselling Team
PEL	Permissible Exposure Limits
PREPP	Post Registration Education and Practice Project
PLUS	Private Line Updating Service

RCN	Royal College of Nursing (London)
RGN	Registered General Nurse
RIDDOR	Reporting of Injuries, Diseases and Dangerous Occurrences Regulations
RNIB	Royal National Institute for the Blind
RoSPA	Royal Society for the Prevention of Accidents
RWL	Recommended Weight Level
SDU	Safety Degree Unit
SME	Small and Medium Enterprises
SOM	Sociey of Occupational Medicine
SPS	Sheltered Placement Schemes
SWORD	Surveillance of Work Related and Occupational Disease
TQM	Total Quality Management
UVL	Ultraviolet Light
WHO	World Health Organization
WRULD	Work Related Upper Limb Disorders

Introduction

OCCUPATIONAL HEALTH: MOVING TOWARDS THE MILLENNIUM

Health, particularly occupational health, concerns everyone – the individual, the family, colleagues, owners, managers, supervisors, unions, governments and governmental organizations. In view of an increasing demand for up-to-date authoritative and validated information it was proposed that a number of specialists should be asked to contribute to a book on related occupational health topics. These specialists readily accepted the challenge and the results are a timely statement on the current movements in occupational health, which in Europe is now driven by European Union legislation.

As an information specialist I know that despite the mountain of occupational health information available, it is difficult to get a state-of-the-art position on the various topics that are covered in this book.

To help the reader *Occupational Health* is divided into four parts. The chapters provide a knowledgeable background to various key subjects and the authors look objectively towards the year 2000, in some cases pointing out the potential problems that will arise if good standards are not secured in the workplace.

Part One provides an introduction to occupational health trends, including not only the *Health of the Nation* implications for the United Kingdom (UK), but also recent progress in developing countries, using Europe as a benchmark. Topics covered are employers' liability, the role of insurance companies/organizations, consultants and liability, and European factors and practices in member states.

Part Two focuses on occupational health in the workplace with chapters on the social aspects of rehabilitation after work related injuries and ill health; the employers role in relation to rehabilitation, alcoholism and drug abuse in the workplace; occupational health diseases, ergonomics, toxicology, hygiene, first aid and paramedics.

Part Three highlights both current and future research; it also looks at the requirements for competent people, determining training needs and delivering training, the need for assessment of capabilities and continuous updating.

Part Four describes the most recent European and worldwide legislation; information sources and services, organizations, publications and computerized sources including online, compact discs and floppy discs. To aid the reader a glossary of acronyms and initials is included.

I hope you, the reader, will find these chapters useful not only in relation to your everyday occupational health problems, but also to give you ideas on how your workplace health standards may be improved.

Sheila Pantry, OBE
Sheffield, October 1994

PART ONE

Worldwide view of occupational health and safety

1

Jukka Takala

BACKGROUND

According to International Labour Office estimates, 120 million accidents occur annually at places of work worldwide. Of these, 210 000 are fatal accidents, meaning that every day more than 500 men or women go to work and never return (Kliesch, 1992). This toll is not widely publicized by the media. The 500 daily fatalities are scattered throughout the world. In contrast, repeated airline accidents killing 500 people daily would receive major attention.

Occupational safety and health may be improved at the national level in essentially four different ways: legislation and regulations, enforcement, information and training, and research. The same methods apply, although somewhat modified, at the company level. Regulations may be equated to company safety policy and guidelines, enforcement to internal inspections, and research could be considered as practical fact-finding at the shop-floor level. Globally, the International Labour Conventions and Recommendations can be considered as binding legislation if ratified by individual states but international enforcement is limited to the follow-up mechanism of those conventions ratified. Table 1.1 lists the conventions and recommendations adopted by the International Labour Organization since 1919.

TRENDS IN GLOBAL DEVELOPMENT

World economic changes will decisively affect conditions of work and environment. Major trends in global change (Rantanen, 1990a; Rantanen, 1990b) encompass:

- a change in production from military to civilian purposes;
- regional concentrations of economic power in three main areas: North America, Europe, and South East Asia;

Table 1.1 List of instruments concerning occupational safety and health and the working environment adopted by the international labour conference since 1919

Year	Convention	Recommendation
1921	13. White Lead (Painting)	
1929	27. Marking of Weight (Packages Transported by Vessels)	
1937	62. Safety Provisions (Building)	53. Safety Provisions (Building)
1946	73. Medical Examinations (Seafarers)	79. Medical Examination of Young Persons
	77. Medical Examination of Young Persons (Industry)	
	78. Medical Examination of Young Persons (Non-industrial Occupations)	
1947	81. Labour Inspection	81. Labour Inspection
		82. Labour Inspection (Mining and Transport)
1949	92. Accommodation of Crews (Revised)	
1953		97. Protection or Workers' Health
1958		105. Ships' Medicine Chests
		106. Medical Advice at Sea
1959	113. Medical Examination (Fishermen)	112. Occupational Health Services
1960	115. Radiation Protection	114. Radiation Protection
1963	119. Guarding of Machinery	118. Guarding of Machinery
1964	120. Hygiene (Commerce and Offices)	120. Hygiene (Commerce and Offices)
	121. Employment Injury Benefits	121. Employment Injury Benefits
1965	124. Medical Examinations of Young Persons (Underground Work)	
1967	127. Maximum Weight	128. Maximum Weight
1969	129. Labour Inspection (Agriculture)	133. Labour Inspection (Agriculture)
1970	133. Accommodation of Crews (Supplementary Provisions)	140. Crew Accommodation (Air Conditioning)
		141. Crew Accommodation (Noise Control)
	134. Prevention of Accidents (Seafarers)	142. Prevention of Accidents (Seafarers)
1971	136. Benzene	144. Benzene
1974	139. Occupational Cancer	147. Occupational Cancer
1977	148. Working Environment (Air Pollution, Noise and Vibration)	156. Working Environment (Air Pollution, Noise and Vibration)

Table 1.1 *Continued*

Year	Convention	Recommendation
1979	152. Occupational Safety and Health (Dock Work)	160. Occupational Safety and Health (Dock Work)
1981	155. Occupational Safety and Health	164. Occupational Safety and Health
1985	161. Occupational Health Services	171. Occupational Health Services
1986	162. Asbestos	172. Asbestos
1987	164. Health Protection and Medical Care (Seafarers)	
1988	167. Safety and Health in Construction	175. Safety and Health in Construction
1990	170. Safety in the use of Chemicals at Work	177. Safety in the Use of Chemicals at Work
1993	174. Prevention of Major Indisutrial Accidents	181. Prevention of Major Industrial Accidents

- continuing rapid technological progress in electronics, information technologies and chemical biotechnologies, contributing to higher productivity and new production methods saving energy and raw materials;
- a need for protection of local and global environment leading to low-waste technologies, recycling and environment-friendly products.

Technological changes in microelectronics increase the capacity and quality of data collection, processing, storage and dissemination. In industrialized countries 30–40% of all workers use computers. The number of robots is increasing by 30–50% per year, and data networks, artificial intelligence and computer-integrated manufacturing systems are being designed and introduced in the production process. As a result, more information on all aspects of production, incorporating safety, is processed and contributes to improved production management.

The development of biotechnologies will influence agriculture, food processing industries, production of pharmaceuticals, hormones, enzymes and biological waste management. Some improvements are expected in safety and health through safer processes, control of emissions and less energy-intensive processes. New hazards, however, may also arise. These may be in the form of genetically manipulated organisms, chemical reactants and new macromolecules, causing new risks of allergy, carcinogenic, teratogenic and mutagenic substances.

Chemical industries continue to grow steadily at a rate of 5–10% per year. Chemicals are nowadays used in all industries and in agriculture.

The transport and use of chemicals will require constant attention with regard to chemical safety in the near future. As both chemicals and workers move from one country to another, the worldwide harmonization of chemical control and information measures becomes essential. This includes the harmonization of classification criteria, standardized labelling systems and chemical safety data sheets.

Service industries will expand more than any other industry. More people will be needed in the health and social services due to an ageing population in industrialized countries. More people in the service sector will be required to master the new technologies.

The world population will continue to grow and the world labour force will double, reaching 5 billion by the year 2050. This means that 2.5 billion new jobs will need to be created in developing countries. The main increase will still be in agriculture, although its relative importance will decrease. This increase in employment also means that the number of fatal and other accidents will double if prevention programmes are not successful. In contrast, trends are opposite in industrialized countries, where population growth may be negative and where workers will be older and therefore less likely to have accidents or be injured.

CHANGES IN OCCUPATIONAL HEALTH AND SAFETY

Information about occupational accidents and diseases is important in order to discover the factors responsible, which can then be subjected to preventive measures and action. Fatal work accidents remain a key indicator of the working conditions and environment. The number of accidents should be compared to the number of active workers exposed to the risks responsible for the fatalities. Making this comparison, the average fatal accident rate using the ILO estimate is in the range 6–7 per 100 000 workers. This rate continues to grow in many developing countries, whereas some industrialized countries have achieved major improvements. Improvements in recording these accidents will lead to more accurate but higher figures in many developing countries and may not reflect true increased rates. However, real increases are also caused by the mechanization and structural changes elevating the number of active workers in the formal employment sector.

Japan reported 5.1 fatalities per 100 000 workers in 1989. France reported a rate of 7.4 fatalities per 100 000 workers (ILO, 1991a). The rates in the Nordic countries are all very similar, the range varying between 3 and 6 per 100 000 (National Board, 1988). The United States reported 8 deaths per 100 000 workers in 1988 which was a drop from 13 deaths per 100 000 in 1980 (US Department of Health, 1989; National Safety Council, 1989). In Sweden and Japan there has been a 70%

reduction of fatal accidents, in Finland – 62%, in the Federal Republic of Germany – 65% during two decades. The annual decline in fatal accident rates in industrialized countries ranges from 2.1% in Belgium 1964–74 to 6.9% in Japan 1968–76 (Pochin, 1987), and in Finland 3.1% 1965–88 (National Board, 1988).

The trends in developing countries have not yet shown similar changes. Countries such as Brazil, Colombia and Mexico, which account for half of the working population of Latin America, report an annual incidence of occupational fatalities in the range of 14 to 27 deaths per 100 000 workers (ILO, 1992). Malaysia reports 29.9 deaths per 100 000 workers (ILO, 1992), Thailand 32.3 (National Institute, 1986) and the Republic of Korea 29.6 deaths per 100 000 workers (Korea Industrial Safety, 1991). Kenya reported 25 and Zimbabwe 27 per 100 000 workers (Takala, 1992).

Although the system of reporting and notification of accidents differs from one country to another and direct comparisons cannot be accurately made, since there is no general agreement as to what the definition of a fatal accident is, one can clearly see the wide gap between industrialized and developing countries.

ACCIDENT RATES IN INDUSTRIES

Agriculture, forestry, mining and construction are industries that continue to lead in the incidence of occupational deaths worldwide. The United States reported that in 1987 the most dangerous field of economic activity was forestry, with 129 deaths per 100 000 workers. The ILO estimates that tropical logging causes 300 deaths per 100 000 workers, i.e. three out of every 1000 workers die annually, or an average of every tenth logger during his working life (ILO, 1991b; ILO, 1991c).

The construction industry continues to be one of the top killers. In the United Kingdom it has been reported that there were more accidents in building operations and engineering construction than in all the manufacturing industries combined. This is even more true in developing countries.

There are, however, certain phenomena that have had a positive impact on reducing the number of occupational deaths from accidents in the 1980s. Deaths of miners due to roof collapses during coal extraction were reduced from 32 to 12 deaths per 100 000 workers as a result of better extraction technology. In industrial countries the number of fatal accidents in forestry and agriculture has fallen, e.g. from 135 in 1966 to fewer than 70 in the 1980s for the United States. The roll-over protection of agricultural tractors has drastically reduced the number of fatal farm tractor accidents (Takala and Kauk, 1983).

A rough estimate is that the number of non-fatal reported accidents (temporary disability of three days or more) is approximately 1000 times higher than that of fatal work accidents. As it is already difficult to compare the national figures for fatal accidents among countries, it is even more complicated for non-fatal work accidents. Differing reporting systems and practices make it practically impossible. However, comparisons from year to year of trends within a country are available. These are declining in many countries, but have reached a plateau in some others (National Board, 1989). Improved intensive care and first aid has influenced the fatal accident figures, but these do not lower all accidents rates.

Accident figures are also affected by many other factors not directly related to the level of safety, such as the intensity of industrial activity (whether an industrial boom or recession) and structural changes. A declining trend is often due to a shift from manufacturing industries – known to be more hazardous – to services, trade and commerce, with their less serious risks. Intensive preventive country programmes have no doubt also had an effect in reducing the number of accidents. This is unfortunately not the case in most developing countries, where the picture is not so clear and where under-reporting and non-coverage by legislation and enforcement is a serious problem.

OCCUPATIONAL DISEASES

In some industrialized countries the number of fatal occupational diseases is quickly rising (Figure 1.1, Finland). Rather than indicating that the working conditions have been rapidly deteriorating, the increasing incidence reflects the fact that occupational diseases are better recognized than before. Particularly, occupational cancer – often caused by asbestos – seems to be better detected than before. However, these new figures are alarmingly high when one takes into account that virtually only one agent (asbestos) caused the rise. Others may still lie undetected. Furthermore, asbestos has been banned or severely restricted in many industrialized countries but is commonly still used in many parts of the world. Occupational diseases are generally poorly recognized in developing countries, only a few diseases are listed in national regulations and these are seldom reported.

There is no similar indicator for work-related diseases. Recognized occupational diseases such as lead poisoning and occupational cancer are only a small part of the total of diseases caused or affected by work. There are many more diseases aggravated by work, a large number of which, such as bronchitis or cardiovascular diseases, are due to multiple factors, some of which are not associated with work. This is one priority field of action in the future within the financial

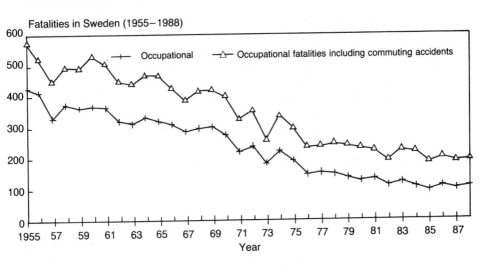

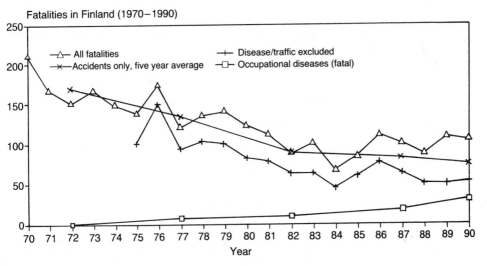

Figure 1.1   Occupational fatalities in Sweden and Finland.

constraints imposed upon us even in the richer parts of the world
(Figure 1.1).

OCCUPATIONAL FATALITIES AND PER CAPITA
GROSS NATIONAL PRODUCT

When comparing the level of economic development measured by the
per capita gross national product (GNP) to fatal accident rates, it is

clearly evident that low productivity is linked to high fatal accident rates. The order is not exactly inverse for several reasons. Empolyment patterns in more and less hazardous industries are not the same. For example, Norway and other Nordic countries have a different structure of economic activities. The current exchange rates, such as the over-valued US dollar at the time of recording in the case of the United States, affect the ratio. Social values and different emphases result in differences in government policies and resources directed for prevention. Finally, free market forces or government-regulated social policies, as in the United States, Japan and most of Europe, also affect the ratio.

Although fatal accident rates are negatively correlated to the gross national product per capita, it is not clear why. An easy hypothesis would be to say that richer countries can afford higher safety standards. But the reverse is as true: no country could demonstrate high per capita GNP with a poor safety record. It may be too simple to state that safety always accompanies productivity, but Figure 1.2 shows that, in general, it does so.

There are certainly safety investments that cannot be justified solely for short-term enterprise-level efficiency reasons. However, apparently lower absence rates and a better motivated and happier workforce that adopts company values and goals as their own will pay in the long term. Four key areas that affect productivity and personal welfare are working conditions, work content, work skills and leadership (Teikari,

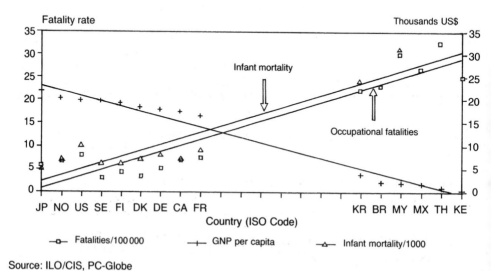

Source: ILO/CIS, PC-Globe

Figure 1.2 Work fatalities, infant mortality, GNP/capita, selected countries.

1989). Highly successful large and small enterprises have, without exception, a better safety record than the average. Conversely, those companies that have a particularly poor safety record will not succeed. Having to avoid hazards at places of work is non-productive and time-consuming and thus lowers the output (Saari, 1986). A major safety disaster, such as the Bhopal accident, will ruin a company's reputation for years or even result in factory closure.

At the national level, a direct positive correlation exists between some public health measures, such as infant mortality or average life expectancy, and fatal occupational accident rates. This correlation is clear and amazingly precise, as can be seen from Figure 1.2. This suggests that a country's health and safety system, policies, practices and attitudes, as well as probably its educational level, all have a positive influence on productivity.

EXPECTED CHANGES IN THE 1990s

Although accidents remain a major problem throughout the world, it is equally important to identify new trends in the field of safety and health. In industrialized countries, a shift of emphasis is to be expected. According to a recent study, and from the international experience, one can predict the following changes:

- occupational stress will increase in importance;
- chemical substances will receive more attention (occupationally and environmentally);
- employment patterns will shift, requiring retraining;
- psychological problems are increasing;
- accidents involving new technologies are increasing;
- noise, physiological and climatic problems and traditional machinery accidents are of less importance (Pröll, 1991).

The basis of these trends should be considered. They are:

- ageing population, early retirement;
- higher demands for productivity, intensive production, pace of work;
- demands for flexibility, self-regulation or deregulation and self-inspection;
- less interest in trade unions;
- higher expectations for job satisfaction, personal health;
- need to know the risks related to work (and private life).

TYPES OF INFORMATION ON OCCUPATIONAL HEALTH

Health and safety information can be classified in many ways, such as statistical figures and descriptive information, reference data and full

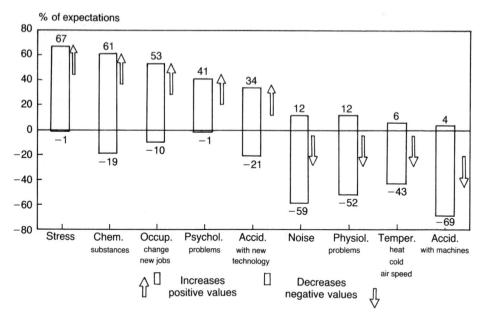

Figure 1.3   Expected changes in the 1990s in industrialized countries (source: Pröll, 1991).

text, or **quantitative** data and **qualitative** data. Information from the system is often expressed in figures, i.e. quantitative, while information to the system is mostly qualitative.

QUANTITATIVE SAFETY INFORMATION

Information in factual, quantitative form is essentially found in figures. It may be measured as nominal values, such as the number of accidents, or in ordinal values indicating priorties. Or it may be expressed in ratios, such as frequency and severity rates of accidents. The real problem is to find criteria for safety effectiveness and some ways to measure it (Tarrants, 1980). Another problem is to design measures which can be both efficient in describing the effectiveness of safety measures as well as understandable to all concerned, in particular to workers and users of chemicals and equipment. If risks are not correctly understood and perceived, one cannot expect rational and safe behaviour either by workers or by management, designers, suppliers and others concerned with safety.

Quantitative risk data is not, in general, well understood. There is broad public confusion about which are the greater hazards and which the smaller, because there is no uniform measure of risk. One of the reasons is that public media do not emphasize continually occurring or even major problems, but tend to highlight sudden and surprising 'shocking' news. Another factor is that processing complex risk information may exceed the cognitive abilities of individuals, so that they rely on heuristics to make these tasks manageable. In general, low risks are overestimated and high risks underestimated (Viscusi and Magat, 1987). This may be understood if we assume that without any information, all risks would be considered as equal. Every piece of information and experience will then partially correct the false risk perception. It has been shown that safety information will influence behaviour. The change in behaviour is influenced not only by the content of this information but also by the form in which it is presented, for example, attractiveness, understandability.

The purpose of any scale to measure safety should be:

(a) to select as targets for prevention those risks that are greatest;
(b) to select as targets those about which it is possible to do something.

In order to understand which hazards are greater than others, we must have a clear, widely understood index, scale or measure of risks (Urquhart and Heilmann, 1984). It would be most logical to start from the fatal accident risk, or other death risks, as information on fatalities deals with major risks and is commonly available.

The most informative ratio scales may be established in several different ways.

1. Perhaps the most commonly used scale, the fatality rate, provides data in the form of death cases divided by 100 000 per unit time. For example, there are 300 fatalities per 100 000 per year in trawling and fishing at sea in the United Kingdom (Pochin, 1987). Tobacco smoking is estimated to cause 170 premature deaths per 100 000 smokers per year in the United States (Urquhart and Heilmann, 1984).
2. The fatal accident frequency rate (FAFR) is the number of fatal accidents occurring in 1000 men in a lifetime working at a particular job (Kletz, 1992). The fatal accident frequency rate was four in the United Kingdom (ca. 1980) in industries and 20 for other accidents, mostly on the road and at home. It was 370 for all diseases. These figures mean that out of 1000 men, four will die at work during their working lifetime, 20 through other accidents and 370 will die from disease, if the UK rates do not change. Kletz also estimates a design value for processes so that they would not increase the average risk. An increase of 1% is hardly likely to cause the worker much concern and an increase of 0.1% certainly should not do so. This gives a design range of 10^{-5} to 10^{-6} per year. The choice of 1000 men is

arbitrary and approximately equivalent to 50 000 man-years or 100 million man-hours. The figures of 1.0 FAFR and 2.0 deaths per 100 000 per year are approximately the same.

3. Risk may be also expressed as shortened life expectancy. Work in a particularly hazardous job may shorten your life from its average expectancy. For example, a man of 20 who works for one year in deep-sea fishing loses 51 days from his life expectancy. However, once he changes his job to a less hazardous one he regains his earlier longer life expectancy as the hazards in deep-sea fishing are acute. The figure 51 days is an average of those few who die early and of many who die old (Urquhart and Heilmann, 1987).

4. Lifetime death rate per 100 000 (or per 1000 or 10 000). This scale is quite close to the FAFR; the working lifetime or work exposure is calculated to be 45 years. In construction industries, the lifetime risk of work-related death per 1000 persons, 1983–84 in the United States was calculated to range from 10.3 to 11.8 (Wrenn, 1987). This would be approximately 23 fatalities per 100 000 workers per year.

5. The unicohort is the smallest group or number of exposed people where a fatality is expected to occur annually. The smaller the unicohort, the greater the risk. A unicohort size of 116 means that one person out of every 116 is expected to be subject to the occurrence, in this case a fatal accident, in any one year. The unicohort size for construction workers in Kenya is 940. That is, in every construction site of more than 940 workers, one can expect one fatal accident once a year. A unicohort may be easily obtained from the fatalities per 100 000 rate by dividing the figure 100 000 by the number of fatalities. That is, the unicohort is the inverse of fatalities per 100 000; in the Kenyan example 100 000/107 = 940 (Urquhart and Heilmann, 1984).

6. The safety-degree scale is based on the concept of unicohort size. The safety-degree unit (SDU) is logarithmic, just as are many other biological and physiological scales. To convert the unicohort size to SDUs, one takes the logarithm (base 10) of the unicohort size: $\log_{10}$ of 940 is 3.0. The safety-degree unit increases when safety itself increases. It normally ranges between values 0 to 10. 'Risk' and 'safety-degree' are semantic inverses of one another (Urquhart and Heilmann, 1984).

7. Chronological age and risk-age conceptualization is based on the difference between average life expectancy and life expectancy in specific circumstances. In risky conditions, the remaining life expectancy is shortened. In essence, the person at risk becomes 'older' than he or she really is. For example, the life-shortening effect of smoking one cigarette is one minute. If you are 33 years old and smoke cigarettes, your smoking decreases your overall degree of

safety by 0.3 SDU, which corresponds to a doubling of your normal, age-related death risk. In terms of the standard life insurance premium table, you are no longer 33, but 40, which is the age at which mortality is double that at age 33.

Most industrialized countries have also established systems for rating less serious accidents. These include the disabling injury frequency rate, the incidence rate (injuries divided by worked man-hours) and serious injury index (Tarrants, 1980). These are excellent indicators within a country but cannot be used for wider comparisons, as recording and reporting systems and practices differ greatly from one country to another.

At the factory level, quantitative information is usually collected in the form of number of accidents, near misses, rates of absenteeism and industrial hygiene measurements. In larger companies or health centres, statistical reports are based on workers' medical records. National databases containing this type of quantitative data are also available (Burns, 1989; British Occupational Hygiene Society, 1988).

Quantitative risk limits

There is no general agreement as to 'how safe is safe' or what risk level should be considered as significant. Risk is the probability of injury, disease or death under specific circumstances. Thus all activities involve risk – eating, drinking, exercising, travelling, working, indeed, anything else. 'Safe' is not equivalent to 'risk free'. While numerous possible 'significant risk' cut-offs might be suggested, there are substantial precedents for adopting lifetime risks of 1 in 1000 for occupational risks and 1 in 100 000 for general population risks as rough 'rules of thumb' regarding significant risk (Wrenn, 1987). The US Occupational Safety and Health Administration (OSHA) the Environmental Protection Agency (EPA) and NCR for radiation protection have all taken the decision that a lifetime risk of 1 in 1000 is a reasonable cut-off point for significant occupational risk. These are based on the levels of risk in 'safe industries', such as occupations in finance, insurance and real estate services, where the lifetime death rate per 1000 varies from 0.8 to 0.9.

This risk estimate has also been a baseline for OSHA to set Permissible Exposure Limits (PEL) for chemicals. The lifetime risk per 1000 recently set as PELs is from 1 to 2 for ethylene oxide, for vinylchloride 4, for asbestos 6.7, etc. The International Council on Radiological Protection (ICRP) has reinforced the same policy and considers the magnitude of radiation risks to the general public in the light of the public acceptance of other risks of everyday life. It has concluded that 'the level of acceptability for fatal risks to the general public is an order of magnitude lower than for occupational risks'. Also, the Ontario Royal Commission and the British Royal Society concluded that a lifetime (general public) risk of 1 in 100 000 does not cause undue concern (Wrenn, 1987).

It is much easier to set limits for occupational risks in conventional industries, where the fatalities are acute, than to set similar benchmarks for ionizing radiation, or carcinogenic substances, or asbestos and other similar hazards which cause delayed effects, which may only be observed after 25, say, years have elapsed. Epidemiological evidence quoted by Doll and Peto (1985) indicates a variation of risk for fatal cancer in textile workers using asbestos with duration of exposure and with age at an exposure level of 0.25 fibres per ml of air, in the order of 20 per 100 000 at risk (Pochin, 1987). Information such as this estimate would be the background for setting exposure limits for non-acute effects.

A voluntary risk is accepted much more easily than an involuntary one such as an occupational risk. The public is willing to accept 'voluntary' risks at roughly a 1000 times greater rate than 'involuntary' risks (Hammer, 1981). According to Viscusi and Magat (1987), people will accept risk that is 10 to 100 fold higher in voluntary activities than they are willing to accept in activities imposed on them. The estimates are not necessarily inconsistent since the range is wide and is affected by a number of factors, such as age, experience, education, length of exposure, financial implications, and income. Risk acceptance varies widely also in selecting an occupation, probably because occupation is a 'voluntary' selection. Furthermore, risk information is normally not available or not properly perceived. The risk in dangerous occupations in Canada ranges from 344/100 000 in mining (cutting and loading) occupations to 146/100 000 in timber cutting and 0.2/100 000 for general office clerks according to Meng (1991).

Because risk acceptance is negatively related to income, higher-income workers should be more likely to regard a job as dangerous, at any given risk level (Viscusi and Magat, 1987). This may be another factor affecting the correlation between the GNP/capita and safety in Figure 1.2. Table 1.2 collects together examples of available quantitative safety information expressed in the various ways described above.

The overall level of acceptance of any given risk depends not only on the probability of undesired effects but also on the frequency of exposure in individual circumstances, as well as on the degree of severity of consequences. There is thus a need to assess these factors all together. A risk score may be established by multiplying the consequences by the exposure and the probability. This score may then be evaluated against a standard scale. A hazard assessment matrix may combine the frequency and severity factors, as explained by Roland and Moriarty (1990). Furthermore the cost-effectiveness of risk reduction measures may be quantitatively assessed and, as a result, a justification factor for different countermeasures may be obtained (Petersen, 1989).

QUALITATIVE HEALTH AND SAFETY INFORMATION

Just as quantitative safety information is necessary to concentrate our efforts on essential safety problems, qualitative information is needed to find practical solutions. By its nature this information cannot be quantitative but is descriptive. It includes legal information, training materials, including audiovisuals, labels, signs and symbols, chemical and technical safety data sheets, standards, codes of practices, text-books, scientific periodical articles, dissertation theses, posters, news-letters, leaflets and so on. The variety of materials makes it much more difficult to classify and subsequently retrieve these materials when needed.

The key issue of safety information is its understandability. Com-prehension requires that information be presented in a way that will be understood by the end user. Language, both everyday and special technical language (jargon), creates, perhaps, the greatest barriers to the global dissemination of safety information.

MEETING THE CHALLENGE

In our joint effort to tackle these common issues, a more coherent and concerted effort is essential. Above all, this is a challenge for us all in view of the constraints we have in material and human resources. To meet this challenge, it has been proposed to further embark on the three visible trends: a long-term strategy to promote roles of social partners; extending protection on a priority basis; and mobilizing local resources. The following three parameters could be used in determin-ing local priority action that should be effective in meeting this challenge while recognizing the resource constraints: first, the need to develop the cooperation of social partners in the assessment and control of workplace risks based on international labour standards; the control should include new methods, such as safety management and internal control; secondly, extending protection to under-served working populations and vulnerable groups where social protection is parti-cularly acute; this relates, in particular, to economies in transition and to developing countries; thirdly, a strategy to mobilize local resources by a variety of measures that complement and support each other;

Table 1.2 Relative risk of fatal accidents in industrial and general environments

Activity or condition	Fatals/100 000 exposed	SDU (Safety Degree Unit)	Unicohort size
All causes, USA	860	2.06	116
All causes, Finland	760	2.12	132
Diseases, UK	740	2.1	140
Cigarette smoking	170	2.8	600
Accidents at construction work			
Thailand	129	2.9	780
Kenya	107	3.0	940
Motorcycling, USA	100	3.0	1 000
All accidents, USA (1969)	60	3.2	1 670
All accidents, Finland (1980)	50	3.3	2 000
Passenger in motor vehicle, USA	17	3.7	6 000
Traffic accidents, Finland (1980)	15	3.8	6 700
Pedestrian, USA	4	4.4	25 000
Bicycling, USA (from whole population)	1	5.0	100 000
Air travel, USA	0.14	5.9	730 000
Accidents at work, Thailand (1984)	32	3.5	3 100
Accidents with agric. tractors (Finland) (estimate per 100 000 users)	32	3.5	3 100
Accidents at work, Kenya (1979)	25	3.6	4 000
Accidents, construction work, Norway	19	3.7	5 300
Accidents, construction work, Finland	16	3.8	6 300
Accidents, construction work, Sweden	8	4.1	12 500
Accidents, construction work, Denmark	8	4.1	12 500
Accidents at work, UK	8	4.1	12 500
Accidents at work, Norway	8	4.1	12 500
Accidents at work, Finland (1977–80)	7	4.2	14 300
Accidents at work, Sweden	4	4.4	25 000
Accidents at work, Denmark	4	4.4	25 000
Accidents at work, whole world, ILO estimate	6	4.2	16 700
All causes, non-smokers, USA, estimate	820	2.1	120
All causes, smokers	1530	1.8	65
All causes, asbestos workers non-smokers	900	2.0	110
All causes, asbestos workers smokers	2460	1.6	40

	Risk per hourly exposure (10^{-6})	Safety Degree Unit	Unicohort size
Asbestos risk for whole population	0.23	5.6	430 000
0–1-year-old children, Finland (1983), infant mortality	700	2.2	140
0–1-year-old children, USA (1983), infant mortality	1100	2.0	90
20-year-old men, USA (1980)	185	2.7	540
20-year-old women, USA (1980)	61	3.2	1 640
40-year-old men, USA (1980)	268	2.6	370
40-year-old women, USA (1980)	149	2.8	670
60-year-old men, USA (1980)	1907	1.7	50
60-year-old women, USA (1980)	958	2.0	105
Coronary heart disease, 55–64-year-old men			
Finland	1030	2.0	97
USA	940	2.0	105
France	200	2.7	500
Coronary heart disease, all males			
Finland (1980)	275	2.6	365
USA (1978)	262	2.6	380
Japan (1979)	40	3.4	2 500
Cancer, Finland (1980)	190	2.7	530
Cerebrovascular diseases, Finland (1980)	120	2.9	830
Poisoning, Finland (1980)	6	4.2	16 700
Drowning, Finland (1980)	3	4.5	33 300
Falls, Finland (1980)	11	4.0	9 100
Falls, USA (1969)	9	4.0	11 100
Fires and hot surfaces, USA (1969)	4	4.4	25 000
Childhood leukaemia caused by an exposure to magnetic fields (for exposed population)	1	5.0	100 000
Electrocution, USA (1969)	0.6	–	–
Machinery, USA (1968)	1	5.0	100 000
Railways, USA (1969)	0.4	5.4	250 000
Coal-based electricity production	0.13	5.9	770 000
Lightning	0.05	6.3	2 mill.
Nuclear power, USA	–	>8.0	>200 mill.

Smoking, hunting and skiing are estimated to be equally dangerous per hourly exposure: 10^{-6} fatalities/person-hour of exposure.

The Safety Degree Unit is a concept describing the relative safety level with simple figures between 0 and 10. It is based on a logarithmic value of the unicohort size.

Unicohort is the smallest group where a fatality will annually occur. The smaller the unicohort, the greater the risk. A unicohort size of 116 means that 1 person out of every 116 will be subject to the occurrence, e.g. fatal accident, in any one year. Unless stated otherwise, risks are calculated for the population as a whole. In other cases, the risk is valid for the exposed group only.

such strategies should rely on efficient and modern information and communication methods.

REFERENCES

British Occupational Hygiene Society Institute of Occupational Hygienists (1988) *Management of occupational hygiene information*. Proceedings of the first UK Conference on Occupational Hygiene Databases, Health and Safety Executive, Sheffield, UK.

Burns, D.K. and Beaumont, P.L. (1989) The HSE National Exposure Database – (NEDB). *The Annals of Occupational Hygiene*, **33**(1), 1–14.

Doll, R. and Peto, J. (1985) *Asbestos; Effects on Health Exposure to Asbestos*, Health and Safety Commission, HSE Books, Sudbury, UK.

Hammer, W. (1981) *Occupational Safety Management and Engineering*, Prentice-Hall, Englewood Cliffs, NJ, USA.

International Labour Office (1991a) *Year Book of Labour Statistics*, ILO, Geneva, p. 1028.

International Labour Office (1991b) Occupational Safety and Health in Forestry. Report on the Industrial Activities' Committee, April 1991, ILO, Geneva.

International Labour Office (1991c) Note on the Proceedings, Forestry and Wood Industry Committee, April 1991, Geneva, pp. 44–5.

International Labour Office (1992) Proceedings of the Regional Latin American and Caribbean Workshop of CIS National Centres and Potential Centres, 10–13 July, 1990, São Paulo. ILO PIACT Report/1990/3, Geneva (in English and Spanish).

Kletz, T.A. (1992) *Hazop and Hazan – Notes on the Identification and Assessment of Hazards*, 3rd edn, The Institution of Chemical Engineers, Warwickshire, UK.

Kliesch, G. (1992) Opening Address. High Level Meeting on Safety and Health Priorities, 29–30 July, 1991, Harare, Zimbabwe. African Safety and Health Project (Training and Information), Information and Training Materials No. 1/92, ILO Geneva, pp. 23–5.

Korea Industrial Safety Corporation (1991) Proceedings of the Technical Seminar, 24th Occupational Safety and Health Convention, 1991, Korea Industrial Safety Corporation, Seoul, Republic of Korea, pp. 495–510 (in Korean).

Meng, R. (1991) How dangerous is work in Canada? Estimates of job-related fatalities in 482 occupations. *Journal of Occupational Medicine*, **33**(10), 1084–90.

National Board of Labour Protection (1989) *Industrial Accidents, Official Statistics in Finland*, Government Printing Centre, Helsinki, Finland, pp. 18–29.

National Institute for the Improvement of Working Conditions and Environment (1986) NICE-Project Final Report, UNDP/ILO Bangkok, ILO Geneva.

National Safety Council (1989) *Accident Facts, 1989*, National Safety Council, Chicago, USA, pp. 2–47.

Petersen, D. (1989) *Techniques of Safety Management, A Systems Approach*, Aloray Inc., New York.

Pochin, E. (1987) *Assessment of Regulation of Risks*. Proceedings of Fibres in Friction Materials Symposium, 1987, The Asbestos Institute, SAE – The Engineering Society for Advancing Mobility, Land, Sea, Air & Space, Friction Materials Standard Institute, Atlantic City, New Jersey, USA.

Pröll, U. (1991) Arbeitsschutzreform und betriebliche Praxis der Arbeitssicherheit (Occupational safety and health reform and enterprise practice in occupational safety). *Die BG, Fachzeitschrift für Arbeitssicherheit und Unfallversicherung,* April, 204–8.

Rantanen, J. (1990a) *New Trends in the Working Life – New Demands for Training.* Proceedings of the Second International Conference on Education and Training in Occupational Health, 6–8 June 1989, Helsinki, Finland. Institute of Occupational Health, Helsinki, pp. 12–23.

Rantanen, J. (1990b) Occupational Health in the Future. International Commission of Occupational Health, Triennial Report 1987–1989, Singapore, pp. 25–9.

Roland, H.E. and Moriarty, B. (1990) *System Safety Engineering and Management,* 2nd edn, John Wiley & Sons Inc., New York.

Saari, J. (ed.) (1986) Työturvallisuuden tehostaminen kokeilututkimusten valossa (Improving Safety Performance: A review of literature on field experiments). *Institute of Occupational Health, Research Report 1986:4,* Helsinki, Finland, pp. 267–83 (in Finnish).

Takala, J. (1992) *Safety and Health Information Systems, Analysis of Local, National and Global Methods.* Tampere University of Technology, Tampere and International Occupational Safety and Health Information Centre, International Labour Office, Geneva.

Takala, J. and Kauko, O. (1983) *Accident Prevention – Results of Safety Activities Carried Out by the Inspectorate.* Proceedings of the 2nd Finnish–Kenyan Symposium on Occupational Safety and Health, Nairobi, Kenya, 1983, National Board of Labour Protection, Tampere, Finland, pp. 192–203.

Tarrants, W.E. (1980) *The Measurement of Safety Performance,* Garland STPM Press, New York and London.

Teikari, V. (1989) Good work contents and skills: A basis for productivity and controlled change, in *Psychological Task Analysis, Design and Training in Computerized Technologies* (eds V. Teikari, W. Hacker and M. Vartiainen), working papers of Otaniemi–Dresden workshop, 1989, Report 113, Industrial Economics and Industrial Psychology, Helsinki University of Technology, Helsinki, Finland, pp. 1–21.

Urquhart, J. and Heilmann, K. (1984) *Risk Watch,* Facts on File Publications, New York, USA.

US Department of Health and Human Services (1989) National Traumatic Occupational Fatalities 1980–1985. NIOSH, Cincinnati, USA, pp. 15–28.

Viscusi, W.K. and Magat, W.A. (1987) *Learning about Risk,* Harvard University Press, Cambridge, MA, USA.

Wrenn, G.C. (1987) *Risk Assessment and the Determination of Significant Risk.* Proceedings of the Fibres in Friction Materials Symposium 1987, The Asbestos Institute, The Engineering Society for Advancing Mobility, Land, Sea, Air & Space, Friction Materials Standard Institute, Atlantic City, New Jersey, USA.

Health concepts 2

Paul Lloyd

The success of a business depends on many factors, not the least of
which is the necessity of maintaining a healthy, happy and productive
workforce. This chapter puts the concept of health into perspective
and focuses on the issues an employer will need to consider.

DEFINING HEALTH

Health is a difficult concept to grasp and the word has a variety of
different meanings. The World Health Organization's definition is 'the
absence of disease or infirmity, a state of bodily, mental and social
wellbeing'. A healthy worker should be able to accomplish the tasks
by which he or she earns a livelihood. The workplace and the operations undertaken in it can adversely affect the health of the worker.
Health cannot be maintained if there are health hazards in the workplace which undermine or destroy the health of workers, such as
noxious fumes, dusts, chemical hazards or poor ergonomic design
leading to musculo-skeletal problems. This is often referred to as the
effects of work on health. Conversely, a person's state of health may
adversely affect his or her work. A high level crane driver may not be
able to continue his occupation if he suffers from blackouts. Such a
person may not only be a danger to himself but to others. It is necessary
to screen potential workers for certain occupations where there is a risk
to the health and safety of other workers or to a wider public.

Not everyone has the same expectations of what is meant by health.
A person confined to a wheelchair having been paralysed from the
waist down may be superbly fit in all other respects and consider him
or herself to be very healthy, as indeed is the case, and may even
participate in the paraplegic olympics. Such a person may also be
able to perform a responsible job provided certain adaptations and

modifications are made to the workplace. The assessment of fitness for work requires an ability on the part of the practitioner to be able to judge health and fitness in relation to the work or proposed occupation. Edwards and McCallum (1988) summarizes general fitness for work in terms of any residual abilities the person may have in relation to the work to be done. This should always be judged with the work in mind and not the pension scheme. A range of medical conditions and virtually all minor ones have no implications for the workplace. Health concepts require that a wider view of health is taken in relation to work and society generally.

Coleman, writing in the foreword of the book by Downie, Fyfe and Tannahill (1993), identifies at least five factors which influence or interact on health. These are:

1. biological factors such as ageing, and genetic changes;
2. lifestyle including behaviour;
3. environment which includes communicable diseases;
4. social and economic factors;
5. use of and access to health services.

The achievement and maintenance of an optimum state of health is therefore not only an individual matter but also a community one. Indeed it has worldwide importance.

HEALTH STRATEGIES GLOBAL AND NATIONAL

The World Health Organization (WHO) set out a global strategy for health for all by the year 2000 (WHO, 1981) at the 32nd World Health Assembly. This was in the form of a resolution endorsing the Report of the International Primary Health Care Conference held in 1978 at Alma Ata (WHO, 1978).

The purpose of this initiative was to enable all people to attain the highest possible level of health so that they are at least capable of working productively and able to enjoy a social life in their own communities. Vast differences exist between the health status of peoples in developed countries and the underdeveloped third world countries, yet each has its problems.

In the United States of America this strategy is summed up in a project known as Healthy People 2000 Promotion (US Department of Health, 1990). This project is designed not only to promote health and prevent disease but to harness professional skill, provide community support and secure individual commitment linked to political will to help people achieve their full potential to lead full and active lives. This strategy also aims to prevent premature death, and disability, help to maintain a healthy environment, and empower people as individuals and in communities to act in order to maintain a maximum level of function.

The WHO produced a total of 38 targets (WHO, 1993) which are being addressed by its European Region and which have been set out to ensure equity in health by reducing existing inequalities between groups within Europe. These targets are summarized in Table 2.1.

Table 2.1 World Health Organization targets: European region. These target statements are based on the WHO European Region's targets

1. Equity in health by improving living and working conditions for all.
2. Adding life to years. To enable people to develop their health potential by making full use of their existing functional capabilities.
3. Health programmes should be set to enable disabled people to have opportunities to develop their full physical, social and economic potential.
4. There should be a 10% increase in the number of years that people live free from major diseases and disability. This is where health promotion initiatives come into their own.
5. This calls for the elimination of specific diseases such as measles, poliomyelitis, diphtheria, and malaria.
6. Life expectancy at birth should be increased to at least 75 years.
7. Infant mortality should drop to lower than 20 per 1000 live births.
8. Calls for a reduction in maternal mortality.
9. To reduce diseases of circulation with a combination of preventive and treatment programmes.
10. To reduce deaths due to cancers by smoking reduction, screening for cervical cancer and screening programmes for other cancers coupled with early treatment and rehabilitation.
11. To reduce accidents in the home, at work or due to traffic. The occupational death rate due to accidents at work to be reduced by 50%.
12. To address the underlying problems causing the rising trend in suicides.
13. To develop healthy public health policies and ensure people at all levels are able to develop healthly lifestyles by being able to contribute to those policies.
14. To enhance the role of family and community in developing healthy lifestyles through closer links locally with social, health and welfare funded programmes.
15. To develop health education programmes at all levels.
16. Set clear targets for positive health behaviour.
17. Set targets to achieve a reduction in health damaging behaviour, e.g. smoking, overuse of alcohol, illicit drugs.
18. To achieve a global health environment.
19. Those risks related to radiations, toxic chemicals, biological agents or harmful consumer goods are monitored and controlled through adequate measures.
20. To ensure the provision of safe drinking water and the removal of the threat to human health of polluted rivers, lakes and seas.
21. To have in place effective monitoring and control arrangements to ensure safe air quality both indoors and outside.

Table 2.1 *Continued*

22. To reduce risk to human health from food contamination and harmful additives.
23. To eliminate major known risks arising from the disposal of hazardous wastes.
24. To provide people throughout the region with the opportunity of living in houses and settlements which are healthy and safe.
25. To provide all people in the region with a healthy and safe working environment. This will mean introducing occupational health services to cover the needs of all workers, and the development of health criteria to protect workers from physical and chemical hazards, the protection of workers and vulnerable groups and the provision of education and information to protect workers.
26. To develop health care systems based on primary care services with secondary and tertiary services providing specialized diagnostic and therapeutic functions which are too specialized for primary health care.
27. To ensure that health care services and resources are distributed according to need.
28. Primary health care services should provide wide ranging services to meet the health promotion, curative, rehabilitative and supportive needs of the population giving special attention to the needs of the vulnerable, high risk and disadvantaged groups in society.
29. To define the roles of health care providers in primary health care to ensure teamwork among health professionals, lay care workers and the communities with which they work.
30. This target seeks to place the control and coordination of health services to the local community in the hands of the primary health care system.
31. Quality care systems should be built into the health care delivery systems in order to measure the effectiveness of health care provision, safety factors, satisfaction levels, and adequacy of care methods.
32. Research strategies need to be in place to foster research into health care delivery and policy development.
33. Health policies and strategies for all should be developed involving all communities and agencies in their development.
34. The managerial process should also allow for the attainment of health for all through adequate planning and resource allocation.
35. To make health information widely available to communities and individuals to assist the planning, monitoring and evaluation of health services and developments.
36. To make adequate provision for sufficient health manpower through the training of health professionals with emphasis on primary health care.
37. In all Member States education should provide personnel in sectors related to health with adequate information on the country's health for all policies and programmes amd their practical application to their own sectors.
38. Formal mechanisms should exist to evaluate the effectiveness of health technologies and their eficiency and safety.

The importance of these 'targets' is to try to redress the burden placed on society of having to look after sick people who consume more and more health care resources and deprive society of potential human development.

Other factors also have to be considered. As the general health of the population improves within Europe there is an increase in the number of people living healthy and fulfilled lives over the age of 65. WHO (1993) projections are that by the year 2000 the population in the European Region under the age of 15 years will have reduced to less than 22% (from 23%) while those over the age of 65 will rise from 11% to over 13%. Not only will there be fewer potential workers in the future to enter the professions such as the caring professions, but there will be an increase in the number of very old people who will ultimately need care and attention. In the USA the number of those over 85 years of age will have increased by about 30% (4.6. million) by the year 2000. The global strategy will call for a partnership between many agencies both statutory and voluntary. Employers will be very much part of this strategy and will have a role to play.

HEALTH TARGETS IN THE UNITED KINGDOM

Since 1948 the National Health Service in the United Kingdom has been based on the concept of a free health service for all from the cradle to the grave. It was a far-seeing welfare concept which was free to all at the point of delivery. Those in employment and the self-employed were expected to pay towards the enormous costs through the Social Security benefit scheme and through prescription charges.

In the early 1990s the government realized that health care for all was consuming more and more resources and their ability to keep funding the health service from taxation was becoming more of a burden. It was generally regarded as a sickness rather than a health service and was best at giving emergency and acute care. A disproportionate amount of resources had been allocated to hospital acute services while the care of the long-term chronic sick and the increasing proportion of elderly people gave rise to new concerns about more equitable allocation of resources. Most importantly, however, was the realization that if efforts were made at government level to focus on prevention of illness and disability in the first place, the burden on the acute and caring services provided in the community could be reduced.

Consequently the five targets initially selected were:

- Coronary heart disease and strokes
- Mental health
- Sexual health, HIV and AIDS

- Cancers
- Accidents.

The thinking was that if these diseases, which were regarded as avoidable, could be reduced, the burden of treatment on the National Health Service could be eased and the quality of life of people extended. The government set out targets to be achieved by the end of the twentieth century.

The task was formidable for it meant trying to persuade people to alter their lifestyles, to get smokers and drinkers to change or moderate their habits and to encourage the obese to exercise and eat more healthy foods; it also meant trying to reduce stress, conflict and anxieties which give rise to so much mental ill health.

The five government targets selected provoked criticism from some quarters including the Royal College of Nursing (1992) which considered that the targets were too narrowly drawn and called for the inclusion of other factors such as the removal of health inequalities, improvement in employment opportunities and the need to tackle poverty. These and other factors in themselves make it difficult for ordinary people to shoulder the entire burden of personal responsibility for improving their own health. Pollution from diesel engines and exhaust emissions from road vehicles is creating new problems which add to the belief that such pollution is causing a dramatic increase in childhood asthma.

The government was, however, conscious that if health for all was to be a reality by the year 2000, everyone including individuals, business, government and health care providers as well as the wider community had a part to play. The burden was to be equally shared. In its strategy the government proposed action on a number of risk factors associated with each target. Each of these targets is considered in turn. Some employers might wish to address these and other health targets in order to safeguard their own interests by ensuring that a healthy workforce is a happy and productive workforce and also to improve employee relations by creating a healthy and safe working environment. With the internal market within the European Union now a reality, increased competition across the borders for skilled labour will emphasize the importance of such health benefits.

Employers also have to safeguard the interests of those of their workers who are pregnant or disabled and the young as well as the older worker. The targets selected below are not directly work related in so far as they could be described as hazards of an occupation, although in the case of cancers they may be. Workplaces with occupational health services are well placed to address these and other health targets as well as to address the more specific workplace health hazards, diseases and accidents.

CORONARY HEART DISEASE AND STROKES

The target is to reduce the death rates from coronary heart disease and strokes among people under 65 in England by 40% by the year 2000. In preventing these diseases the strategies would also help to prevent other diseases, which is why this is a prime target, and it is one which could be met by changes in personal lifestyle behaviour.

The accepted causes of coronary heart disease and strokes could be readily addressed in the workplace with its 'captive' population. These contributory factors are generally thought to be:

- Smoking
- Obesity and lack of exercise
- Alcohol consumption
- Stress
- High blood pressure
- Raised blood cholesterol levels.

The opportunity should be taken to set up policies and procedures for identifying these risk factors and addressing them. This would mean encouraging healthy eating, tackling alcohol-related problems and giving workers the opportunities to increase the amount of physical exercise they take, which is known to increase life expectancy. Lifestyle counselling is also important if the strategy is to succeed.

Lack of physical exercise is probably the most significant trigger leading to coronary heart disease. This is brought about by a number of factors such as lack of competitive sports in school, and children choosing to spend most of their free time either watching television or playing computer games. A sedentary occupation, lack of recreational facilities in the workplace or neighbourhood and a lack of disposable income or incentive to exercise are all factors compounding the problem.

Greater efforts need to be made both in the workplace and in the community to provide the opportunities and incentives to promote regular exercise. Employers could consider providing in-house facilities or enter into negotiation with local community resources to enable workers to take advantage of subsidised schemes and facilities such as the use of swimming pools and recreational and sports facilities.

The coronary heart disease target provides opportunities to raise awareness of the issues through various strategies such as the development of policies governing alcohol consumption in the workplace, the introduction of healthy eating options in works canteens, closer monitoring of other risk factors such as high blood cholesterol levels, and blood pressure screening by the occupational health service.

Assistance for employees does not only come from in-house occupational health schemes but also from government agencies such as the

Look After Your Heart Workplace Programme administered by the Health Education Authority in England and Wales. This is a statutory body funded by central government with local offices and officials who provide information and action plans on smoking cessation, healthy eating and physical activity on request to workplaces.

The number of employees able to take advantage of such schemes is higher in the larger organizations which usually have an occupational health service, whereas the small organizations normally do not.

MENTAL ILL HEALTH

Stress is considered to be a problem especially in industry. No particular target has been set because of the lack of quantifiable data but mental illness accounts for 14% of certified sickness absence in England (Department of Health, 1992). In the competitive world of industry and commerce and, increasingly, in the caring sector, the pressures on individuals to rise to the challenges of work are enormous. Frequently work overload is a contributory factor to the development of milder forms of mental illness. This is particularly true of nursing where increased levels of sickness absence among nurses has been attributed to work overload and burn-out (Seccombe and Buchan, 1993). Depression is the most common of these disorders. In the USA depression affects 5% of the adult population at any one time (United States Department of Health, 1990). Suicides among the young present the greatest challenge to the policy. There were 5567 deaths in 1991 in England from suicide (Department of Health, 1992).

This topic is of particular concern to industry because of the many causal factors which give rise to these problems in the modern industrial environment. The problem can often pass undetected because there is no strategy to deal with it. The *Health of the Nation Workplace Task Force Report* (1994) recommends that employers should build into their workplace health policy a mental health strategy so that through better education of management and staff a positive attitude is developed. This should bring the following benefits:

- dissemination of stress management techniques;
- improved support for employees;
- help in decreasing the stigma attached to mental illness.

In a report on stress research and management Cox (1993) concluded that there was insufficient knowledge available to support legislation to control stress in the workplace but he favours a European general framework on managing stress at work to set minimum acceptable exposure levels to stress-producing hazards.

He also argues that primary prevention at the organizational level, such as a control cycle similar to the Management of Health and Safety at Work Directive, is the most promising area of activity.

SEXUAL HEALTH AND AIDS

Other targets such as sexual health and AIDS may not be regarded by employers as being of relevance to workplace health promotion strategies. Only 9% of all workplaces surveyed by the Workplace Task Force (The Health of the Nation Workplace Task Force, 1994) addressed this problem.

Some employers have become too concerned about the impact of AIDS on their workforce. Occupational health professionals are not expected to enquire into an individual's sexual orientation or habits, and any specific questions about HIV or AIDS status are definitely ruled out of order. Yet some employers insist that such questions and enquiries be made, and the applicant is sometimes asked to sign a statement verifying the truthfulness of the answers given. This approach raises serious professional difficulties for the occupational health nurse or doctor conducting a health interview. Only with the informed and written consent of the individual to whom the information relates may the nurse or doctor disclose it to a third party.

This is not to underestimate the seriousness of HIV infection or its consequences. The concern of occupational health is therefore to reinforce the messages of prevention as far as possible by way of talks, video presentations and leaflets. There is every reason why nurses should attend special AIDS counselling courses; this is especially important when the occupational health nurse is taken into the confidence of a person who has tested positively for HIV or who admits to having an AIDS related disease. In a health promotion setting it is important for the nurse to learn how to get the right messages across, especially to the young. Precautions at work should include advice related to first aid and blood contact.

CANCERS

Targets have been set for cervical, skin, lung and breast cancers. About 80% of lung cancers are linked to tobacco smoke. The target is to reduce lung cancer deaths in the under 75 year old population by 30% in men and 15% in women. In order to achieve this target there will be a parallel need to reduce cigarette consumption by at least 40% by the year 2000.

The UK government imposes heavy tax duties on cigarette manufacturers and has not banned cigarette advertising outright although it requires a serious health warning to appear on every cigarette packet and is seeking legislation to impose a ban on cigarette advertising within one mile of any school. The advertising agencies complain that this is tantamount to a complete ban on cigarette advertising if it succeeds. This is a typical moral dilemma. The RCN, in its evidence on the Health of the Nation (Royal College of Nursing, 1992), was critical of the government for allowing the tobacco industry to advertise a dangerous drug with very limited restrictions despite the effects of this advertising on the numbers of women and young girls taking up the smoking habit. The RCN called for incentives by government to attract employers to make more workplaces and public areas smoke free. Even the Pentagon in the USA is seeking a ban on cigarette smoking in all its military establishments throughout the world.

The Health of the Nation Workplace Task Force (1994) reported that the smoking cessation target had been well addressed and much significant work had been done. For example, 31% of workplaces in England had addressed smoking as a risk factor. When this figure is compared to the size of the undertaking according to the number of workers, 30% of the workplaces with fewer than 24 workers had no-smoking policies in place, whereas 81% of the larger organizations with over 500 employees had no-smoking policies.

As far as cervical and breast screening is concerned national screening programmes are in operation. Only a small proportion of workplaces appear to support cancer screening programmes at work (3%). Employers are encouraged to persuade women to take full advantage of screening programmes by making facilities for screening available on site or allowing women time to attend for screening appointments. It is vital that women are allowed to follow up positive findings and occupational health services should have arrangements in place for time off for such matters if in-house arrangements cannot be made. The availability of health promotion material at work is an essential aspect of this programme.

ACCIDENTS

According to the Commission of the European Communities (1994) about 8000 people die each year from accidents at work out of a total of 120 million workers. About 10 million workers are victims of accidents or occupational diseases each year.

Accidental death and injury is a serious problem among the young, homicide and violence being the most common cause of death among those under 30 years of age. Accidents arise in the home, on the roads, and at work. Motor vehicle crashes account for approximately one half of deaths from unintentional injuries in the USA. Existing health and safety legislation has had an impact on the rate of occupational accidents along with improved manufacturing technologies and a decline in the number of more hazardous industries such as coal mining and steel manufacture. Accidental injury from manual handling and repetitive strain injury are increasing, especially among nurses who handle and lift patients. It is estimated (Seccombe and Ball, 1992) that in 1990 in the United Kingdom almost 60 million working days were lost due to back pain and that nurses suffered more and had more absence due to this condition than any other group of workers in the United Kingdom.

Targets aim to reduce the death rate for children under 15 years by at least 33% by 2005, and to reduce death rates due to accidents among the under 25 year old population by at least 25% by 2005.

EUROPEAN INFLUENCES ON HEALTH AT WORK

The effects of European and domestic legislation have brought the risk factors associated with workplace ill health under better control. The influence of European directives followed by national legislation such as the Ionising Radiations Regulations 1985, the Control of Substances Hazardous to Health Regulations 1988 and the Manual Handling Operations Regulations 1992 in the United Kingdom has forced a greater awareness on employers of their responsibilities to ensure a safe and healthy place of work, safe systems of work and improved risk management and assessment procedures.

The impact these regulations have had on practice has yet to be fully evaluated. It is the intention of the European Union to review and consolidate its directives on health and safety legislation and ensure that Member States are implementing these through national legislation (Commission of the European Communities, 1994). In some cases directives may need to be brought up to date to reflect advances in technological progress, new knowledge and risks, particularly those arising from toxic substances, carcinogens and harmful agents.

The European Union is also concerned to ensure that its health and safety directives are compatible with international measures for health and safety so as to permit fair competition and trade in world markets and enable free trade between the European Union and the rest of the world.

In this respect the International Labour Office (ILO) Convention and Recommendation on Occupational Health Services will still have an influence to bear. The Convention 161 and Recommendation 171 on the Organization of Occupational Health Services is waiting in the wings for governments to ratify. There are signs that this matter is on the agenda of the Commission of the European Union which has indicated its wish to work in closer harmony with the ILO, the WHO and the United Nations, in order to work towards closer coordination and effectiveness in such matters as the environment and health and safety at work with more emphasis on joint activities. In the meantime the development of occupational health services will remain an employer option, certainly in the United Kingdom, with resultant vast differences in the availability and quality of such services.

HEALTH PROMOTION STRATEGIES

The WHO believes that the Health for All targets are best delivered by the primary health care team. In the United Kingdom such teams have been organized within and focused on the general practitioner service with input from nurses working in community practice. This includes nurses who have completed specialist preparation in the nursing care of adults, general nursing care of children, nursing the mentally ill and nursing the mentally disabled, contributing to the promotion of community health, child protection and health maintenance and the nursing care of employees within the workplace (this relates to the practice of occupational health nursing).

Although occupational health (OH) nursing is included in the primary care team as part of public health nursing, in practice there is no formal arrangement to link OH nurses to primary health care services. Local arrangements are often developed on a voluntary basis and there have been examples of good cooperation between occupational health nurses, doctors and local general practitioner services.

The employer who does not have an occupational health service may enter into an arrangement with local general practices to buy in the services of a doctor. Unless the general practice doctor (GP) has had some training in occupational medicine and the practice nurse some training in occupational health nursing the perceived benefits may be limited.

The Health and Safety Commission (Health and Safety Executive, 1992) has gone to considerable lengths to inform general practice doctors and their nursing staff about the effects of work on health and health on work. Advice offered includes alerting them to a number of work related health issues which could usefully be integrated into the general practice health promotion programmes. Examples include:

- raising awareness of skin care;
- recognizing the synergistic risk of smoking and harmful dusts and fumes;
- coping with stress;
- thinking positively about getting back to work.

In relating occupation to disease patterns a European Commission survey (Commission of the European Communities, 1993) was con-

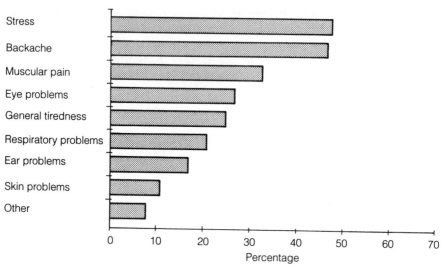

Figure 2.1 Self-reported factors affecting work.

ducted among the Member States to find out what concerns workers had about their own safety and health at work. The chart indicates that stress and backache were the most commonly reported conditions.

Another survey, conducted by the Health and Safety Executive in England and Wales in 1990, gave new information on the extent of ill health in particular occupations (Hodgson *et al.*, 1993). Adults were asked if they had suffered from any illness which they thought had been caused by or made worse by work. Not surprisingly musculo-skeletal conditions were the most commonly reported work related health problem for both manual and non-manual occupations. Some occupations such as teaching had higher than average risks (stress and depression caused by work); the reporting by clerical workers of headache and eyestrain caused by work was twice the average of that reported by other occupations.

If general practitioners and practice nurses are to become more involved with workplace health issues they need to have their level of awareness of work related health issues raised so that they are in a better position to respond to the challenges. There are several good reasons for this. The general practitioner in the United Kingdom has the overall responsibility to provide medical care for his or her patients whether in employment or not. If they have jobs to go to, many of these patients may not have the benefit of an occupational health service at their place of work. There are also some occupational diseases which the general practitioner has to report to the Health and Safety Executive and these must be recognized. If the GP is aware of patients' occupations he or she is in a better position to respond positively to their health educaton needs. Another significant requirement placed upon a GP is that employers can request a medical report to be used for employment purposes. This is intended to give an opinion about whether a person is fit to do a particular job or not. It would be extremely difficult for a GP to be able to make such an evaluation if he or she is unaware of what that job requires in terms of physical or mental demands.

To address this problem, the Health and Safety Executive (Griffin, 1992) recommended that:

- educational establishments introduce occupational health awareness into the nurse practice courses;
- closer cooperation should be fostered between occupational health nurses and practice nurses to improve and exchange both experience and knowledge;
- further study should be undertaken to define the extent of general practitioners' involvement in and knowledge of occupational health matters.

The rationale behind these recommendations is that because occupational health services are not widely available these measures are necessary to raise awareness about occupational health concerns.

Employers first and foremost are concerned with meeting their statutory responsibilities to comply with health and safety legislation. Once these responsibilities have been addressed, employers are more likely to be concerned about health issues which might not be *Health of the Nation* targets but which cause them considerable concern. Back pain and repetitive strain injury serve as good examples.

DELIVERING THE HEALTH MESSAGES

Employers are also looking for cost benefits from addressing health issues at work. How effective are health interventions and how can benefits be measured? These questions are not easy to answer because any preventive health programme cannot be precisely costed although it is possible to make assumptions. A good example, quoted by Sir Duncan Nichol when addressing a conference recently (Cassidy, 1994), is figures from the Taunton Cider Company's Health at Work Programme. These showed a reduction in absenteeism of 21% over 10 years, a reduction in the accident rate of 23% and that time off work due to back related conditions had been cut by 95%. This latter success was attributed to the organization employing a physical therapist to attend to back pain sufferers on the premises.

The methods of putting health messages across to workers differ. In some cases health notices are placed on notice boards and changed frequently, or health advice leaflets may be put into pay packets, or made available in the canteen or at some other strategic point and changed frequently to keep interest alive. In other instances the workers may be expected to attend a formal lecture and perhaps a demonstration. A third example is when there is a one to one counselling relationship between a health professional and a worker. A good example of this is when an occupational health nurse or doctor sees an employee either during a routine visit to the work site or during a treatment or counselling session in the occupational health centre. In this setting it is possible to discuss a problem and agree a solution, and this is when health advice may be more readily accepted.

In addition to this type of approach employers may agree to the organization of special arrangements related to health issues in the workplace, such as health screening for breast or cervical cancer, well man and woman clinics, antenatal clinics, access to counselling by an independent and qualified counsellor on a confidential basis, or health assessments before transfer to other types of work.

In order to be effective it is necessary to plan how health messages and targets are to be presented to workers. It is also important to have some way of measuring the benefits, if any, which result from these initiatives.

Caraher (1994) examines how health promotion models are used in practice. He suggests that nurses should develop a body of expertise in health promotion because they are closer to the client and are ideally placed to do so. Occupational health nurses have always seen this as an inherent part of their duty of care to workers. Health promotion is not simply a matter of imparting knowledge with the nurse as teacher and the worker as pupil.

In the 1960s and 70s there was an overconcentration on the 'victim blaming' approach where the worker was blamed for being overweight or smoking when he or she became ill. It is of little use blaming someone with heart disease who is overweight and smokes unless the wider social factors which often govern peoples lives are also addressed. Hence individuals should not have to bear the entire blame for their own ill health. In any event people often have to cope with different and sometimes conflicting advice provided by health professionals, scientists and researchers. Hence they do not know what to do for the best, or which piece of advice to accept or reject, e.g. is butter good or bad for you?

Caraher (1994) suggests that health promotion models in current use raise concerns because:

- they tend to focus on the skills needed by the nurse to be more effective and efficient;
- the client's socioeconomic factors are seen as of no consequence to the model;
- models which do not question the contribution and role of the nurse are inadequate;
- models need to acknowledge power and control in any health promotion encounter;
- current emphasis in the National Health Service is on the achievement of targets, not with healthy individuals as the objective but as a means to an end.

Therefore the role or the nurse in getting health messages across is of paramount importance. Nurses who have taken a degree or diploma in Occupational Health Nursing are well founded in the required skills of communicator, advocate, and counsellor to the client group although the nurse needs to continue to develop and expand his/her skills in this area.

Health promotion, whether it is undertaken by nurse or doctor, needs to take account of the wider social and political dimensions when health advice is proferred to workers. Any developments and successes in this area also need to be based on sound data collection and surveillance systems. Health authorities are obliged to collect and analyse such data in respect of the populations within their catchment areas. Occupational health services also need to collect baseline data on disease patterns, mortality, disabilities, injuries arising at work or elsewhere among workers (Webb *et al.*, 1988), ill health reports, sickness absence records and the diagnosis of sickness absences.

Employers are more likely to promote health awareness messages if they can see tangible benefits to them from doing so. It is therefore necessary to establish a baseline against which success or otherwise can be measured. Data should be collected, for instance, on sickness absence, accidents and reduced staff turnover. If these figures show an improvement it is also highly likely that there will be an increase in productivity. Unfortunately there is no way to research this data without other factors complicating it. Examples include factors having no direct bearing on work such as lifestyle, environment, and social relationships.

Employers who have set up occupational health services are not always clear about the benefits they want or can expect from such services. Put at its simplest level an employer may see a nurse as

Table 2.2 Summary of process of evaluation

Main actions	Associated actions	Comments
Step 1: Clarify aims and objectives of the proposed health promotion progrogramme	Get people on board. Set up an evaluation group. Check out what the real health problem is. Establish baseline information.	The importance of spending time on this ground work cannot be overemphasized. Involvement of the right people will ensure commitment, use of information generated and a good response to any questionnaires. The evaluation group (minimum of three) should reflect the range of interests. Proper clarification makes the evaluation straightforward.
Step 2: Design the framework of re-evaluation and decide what questions you want to ask	Decide what the purpose of the evaluation is and who is going to use the information. Decide what useful questions to ask in relation to achieving aims and objectives. Decide from whom are you going to collect it. Decide if you want process as well as outcome information.	Do this before you decide what measures to use. If the objectives have been stated clearly this should be relatively easy. Make sure you are clear who the evaluation is for. This affects what questions are asked. The main aim is to see whether the activities in the programme resulted in the stated objectives. Try to look at process as well as outcome.
Step 3: Design the framework for evaluation and decide how you are going to measure change	Decide what you are going to measure and which methods you are going to use. Decide on sample size and target population. Decide when you are going to collect the information.	Good measurement depends on being clear on the issues. Method should be appropriate to the questions and need not be numbers. Be realistic and honest about limitations of time and money.

Step 4: collect the data	Make sure data collection is unobtrusive and does not add to people's workload or if it does that they can see the value of doing it. Make sure people are still on board. Keep people informed by regular feedback. Remember data is not information.	There will be problems of confidentiality and bias. Most common bias is in self reported behaviours. Problems are fewer if everyone has been involved. Participation is a key.
Step 5: Evaluate the results to determine effectiveness of programme	Interpret data in association with evaluation group. Compare what actually happened with what you expected. Remember numbers are only indicators of what the world is like.	Data is not information until it has been interpreted. This is best done as a collaborative process so people are clear how the results were obtained. Do not forget the value of 'soft' information and remember some health changes take time to be revealed.
Step 6: Make recommendations	Clarify what is useful. Cover practical changes for immediate implementation. Include the costs and benefits of not implementing. Challenge existing beliefs. Look at longer term changes that may not yet be visible.	If people have been involved in the process they will already be committed to acting on the findings and be receptive to results.

Table compiled by Dugdill and Springett (1994), Liverpool John Moores University, for Health of the Nation Workplace Task Force.

providing a first aid treatment service for people at work, and any determined attempts that nurse may make, especially in a small organization, to enlarge on this role, even by taking further education in his/her own time, may often be frustrated by the employer who may fail to appreciate the benefit to the organization of an expanded role for the nurse with this specialist education and may see such further education as largely irrelevant to the business.

However in the United Kingdom this scenario is set to change with the reform of post basic nurse education and the concept of the specialist community nurse (occupational health) (United Kingdom Central Council for Nursing, Midwifery and Health Visiting, 1994) fulfilling a role which can only be held by a nurse having undergone such additional specialist education.

At the other extreme the occupational health services with teams of qualified occupational health nurses and doctors and other professionals such as hygienists, may be fully engaged in providing a comprehensive service covering every aspect of occupational health. In most cases the level of provision is a compromise between these two extremes, tailored to meet statutory requirements, immediate hazards to the health of workers and the agreed preferences of the occupational health providers and employers. There is therefore always a potential for conflict as the expectations of the different parties may not coincide.

The maintenance of the health of workers is one example. The occupational health nurse may be just as concerned about the number of people who smoke as he or she would be about the levels of noxious fumes in a particular works department. The employer, on the other hand, may consider that the occupational health nurse (the health expert) should be concentrating on something else entirely and that may not even be related to health at all.

Dorward (1993) found that there are marked differences of emphasis with regard to the perceptions managers have about the role and continuing education needs of the occupational health nurses that they manage. Nurse managers saw the occupational health nurse as provider of a comprehensive, preventive and supportive service which included health promotion, environmental monitoring, emergency care, counselling and rehabilitation of the recovered employee. On the other hand, if the manager was a physician the expectation was that the occupational health nurse would promote health, and provide counselling and first aid, while the lay manager (examples being personnel managers, some executive managers, safety adviser or training officer) saw the occupational health nurse as a provider of treatment for sick or injured employees.

It is interesting that in the area of health promotion both nurse and physician manager saw the nurse as the natural health promoter and organizer of such activity, whereas lay managers saw the nurse's role in this area as being targeted towards specific objectives, such as AIDS, well woman clinics, alcohol, drugs, diet, exercise, screening, organizer of health fairs, and liaison with outside bodies concerned with health issues.

This survey showed that not only was the occupational health nurse involved in a variety of ways in health issues at work but other groups of people were also involved. Examples included training officers, physicians, safety personnel, physiotherapists and outside bodies.

To underpin this point the European Foundation for the Improvement of Living and Working Conditions (personal communication) is developing a specification for training in workplace health promotion. This organization is surveying organizations in the European Union to establish what training courses in health promotion exist in each country and the content of such courses. Their target group for the development of such a specification, which they do not see as primarily a medical activity, includes occupational health doctors, nurses, safety practitioners, human resource personnel, occupational hygienists, health and safety representatives, trade union officials and other professions able or willing to set up health promotion activities within organizations. The inclusion of such groups is reflected in the scope of health promotion. The concept is to include any activity which sets out to improve the physical, psychological and social environment of work, even changing shift patterns if it can be shown to have a beneficial effect on health.

This holistic approach to health, which raises questions about who delivers the health messages or develops health policies in the workplace, is an important development which empowers people and communities to take responsibility for safeguarding and improving their own health and is entirely in keeping with the WHO health targets.

The Wellness Forum, which started in North America, has now been established in the United Kingdom. It is employer led and aims to involve the largest organizations in a wellness movement to promote good health among workers. It has the support of some of the largest UK organizations. It aims to encourage the development of health strategies in the workplace and exchange information among its members on good practice. It provides a platform for occupational health professionals, personnel and welfare officers, managers and other experts to come together and develop ideas to promote wellness among workers. The bottom line is good health is good for business.

EVALUATING HEALTH MESSAGES

In practice there may be considerable health promotion activity going on in any particular setting but is it having any effect? Are people changing behaviour and adopting healthier lifestyles, are improvements being made to workplace environments, and is the working population healthier as a result? It will not be possible to find out unless a strategy has been developed to measure what has been achieved.

The holistic approach to health promotion where almost everyone in a position of influence over others can be viewed as a health promoter does not necessarily produce a leader capable of identifying all the issues and evaluating the outcome of the interventions.

In this context the influence of the occupational health nurse is of paramount importance as the nurse provides the focus for action, the caring professional with education in health sciences who is capable of organizing health-related activity through the sharing of knowledge with the client. It requires the nurse to act as a catalyst for change by engaging in reflective practice.

Driscoll (1994) points out the new generation nursing courses where reflective practice – 'the thinking, questioning professional' – has now taken over from the 'doers' in nursing, when 'doing' was a highly valued quality in nursing circles. Driscoll therefore offers a framework for retrospective structured practice, an evaluation process which ensures that routine activities are now taken for granted. These stages can be summed up as follows:

- returning to the situation;
- understanding the context;
- modifying future outcomes.

Guidelines for the evaluation of health promotion programmes in the workplace have been produced by Dugdill and Springett (1994) following an extensive literature search (Table 2.2). Their conclusions are that current research studies conducted in North America, Japan, and Scandinavia show that workers are more productive, experience fewer accidents and take less time off work when health promotion programmes have been introduced. They also found that the most successful programmes are the ones where workers themselves have been involved in deciding what programme to introduce and in implementing and evaluating them. They describe Japan as having the highest worker productivity rates in the world with more money spent per head than any other country on health promotion programmes.

Ewles and Simnett (1992) suggest five approaches to health promotion which can be described thus.

1. The medical approach which depends on patient compliance with preventive medical procedures.
2. Behavioural change where individual behaviour is conducive to change by encouraging the adaptation of a healthier lifestyle.
3. Educational approach with individuals having the knowledge and understanding to be able to make well-informed decisions and act upon them. It is the health promoter's responsibility to identify the educational content.
4. The client centred approach, working with clients on their own terms so that clients are equals who are able to set the agenda and have self-empowerment.
5. Societal change where the physical and social environment enables choices to be made between healthier lifestyles, based upon political and social action to change the physical and social environment.

CONCLUSIONS

Health maintenance is a complex issue affecting individuals, communities, employers, health care agencies, governments and international agencies. The WHO targets provide a focus for action and the evidence is that these targets are being addressed in a variety of ways with variable success. There are opportunities for occupational health practitioners and their employers to do more in promoting health and evaluating the outcome of their endeavours. More research is needed into how organizations address health promotion in the workplace and with what benefits. There is a need for more guidance for employers and their staff on health concepts in the workplace. Employers who have not so far seen the need for occupational health advice should reconsider and avail themselves of the opportunities to explore the issues raised in this chapter.

REFERENCES

Caraher, M. (1994) Health promotion time for an audit. *Nursing Standard*, 8(20), 32–5.

Cassidy, J. (1994) NHS should look to industry to improve health at work. *Nursing Times*, 2 February, 90(5), 7.

Commission of the European Communities (1993) *General practitioners and occupational diseases*. Office of Official Publications, Luxembourg.

Commission of the European Communities (1994) General Framework for action in the field of safety, hygiene and health protection at work (1994–2000). CEC/V/F/LUX/43/93, Office of Official Publications, Luxembourg.

Cox, T. (1993) Stress research and stress management: putting theory to work. *Health and Safety Executive Contract Research Report No. 61*, HSE Books, Sudbury, UK.

Department of Health (1992) *The Health of the Nation: a strategy for health in England* (Cm 1986), HMSO, London.

Dorward, A.L. (1993) Managers' perceptions of the role and educational needs of occupational health nurses. *Health and Safety Executive Research Paper 34*, HSE Books, Sudbury, UK.

Downie, R.S., Fyfe, C. and Tannahill, A. (1993) *Health promotion models and values*, Oxford University Press, UK.

Driscoll, J. (1994) Reflective practice for practise. *Senior Nurse* 25(7), 47–50.

Dugdill, L. and Springett, J. (1994) The evaluation of workplace health promotion programmes: a brief review of literature. *Health of the Nation Workplace Task Force Report*, Liverpool John Moores University, UK.

Edwards, F.C. and McCallum, R.I. (1988) *Fitness for work*, Oxford University Press, UK.

Ewles, L. and Simnett, I. (1992) *Promoting health – a practical guide*, Scutari Press, London, UK.

Griffin, N. (1992) Occupational health advice as part of primary health care nursing. *Health and Safety Executive Research Paper 30*, HSE Books, Sudbury, UK.

Health and Safety Executive (1992) *Your patients and their work: an introduction to occupational health for family doctors*, HSE Books, Sudbury, UK.

Hodgson, J.T., Jones, J.R., Elliott, R.C. and Osman J. (1993) Self reported work-related illness: results from a Trailer Questionnaire on the 1990 Labour Force Survey in England and Wales. *Health and Safety Executive Research Paper 33*, HSE Books, Sudbury, UK.

Royal College of Nursing (1992) *A Response to the Health of the Nation*. (Strategy for England), Royal College of Nursing, London.

Seccombe, I. and Ball, J. (1992) Back injured nurses: a profile. A Discussion Paper for the Royal College of Nursing, Institute of Manpower Studies, University of Sussex.

Seccombe, I. and Buchan, J. (1993) Absent nurses: the costs and consequences. *Institute of Manpower Studies Report No. 250*, Institute of Manpower Studies, University of Sussex.

United Kingdom Central Council for Nursing, Midwifery and Health Visiting (1994) *The future of professional practice – the council's standards for education and practice following registration*, United Kingdom Central Council for Nursing, Midwifery and Health Visiting.

United States Department of Health and Human Sciences Public Health Service (1990) *Healthy People, National Health Promotion and Disease Prevention Objectives*, Department of Health and Human Services, Washington, DC.

Webb, A., Schilling, R., Jacobson, R. and Babb P. (1988). Health at Work. *Health Education Authority Research Report No. 22*, London, UK.

World Health Organization Alma Ata (1978) *Primary Health Care*.

World Health Organization (1981) *Global Strategy for Health For All by the Year 2000*.

World Health Organization Regional Office Europe (1993) *Health for all targets: health policy for Europe*.

Insurance and liability

3

Terry ap Hywel

This chapter looks first at the legal liability on employers to pay compensation to workers who have suffered disease or ill health as a result of their work. This liability in the UK and many other countries is based on the tort system that requires negligence or fault on the part of someone to be proved.

The next part discusses insurance to meet claims made against employers who are proved to be legally liable for compensation under the tort system. Some notes on the UK Social Security benefit system and other countries' workers' compensation schemes are also provided.

The final part deals with the liability of consultants in the occupational health field with comments on professional indemnity insurance. Some practical suggestions are made to help occupational health consultants provide effective assistance to their insurers when dealing with any claims made against them.

LEGAL LIABILITY

The subject of insurance for the payment of damages to a worker who suffers disease and ill health is linked in the UK and in most other countries with the legal duties of the employer or possibly another person, to consider the health and safety of people who could be affected by their actions or failure to act. In other words, insurers will not normally automatically pay compensation to a worker who suffers some disease or ill health; the worker must be able to show that his or her condition resulted from some failure of someone to comply with a legal duty. This situation often results in lengthy delays and complaints that insurers are heartless and unfeeling!

To understand the insurance aspect it is therefore necessary to discuss the legal aspect of employers' liability for the payment of damages for disease and ill health. The following notes discuss this topic from the viewpoint of the English legal system. Many other countries' legal systems are similar, particularly those of countries whose legal systems are based on a common law approach; they will however differ in detail as their law has been shaped by various individual national and political factors. These notes do not offer a full explanation of the law – further reading is recommended if clarification is required on any point (Munkman, 1990). In any case the law is constantly changing and being refined so this chapter has been written with the intention of outlining basic principles only in the hope that it will remain valid for some time to come.

An employer may incur liability at **common law** or for **breach of statutory duty**. Each of these is discussed below. Usually when a claim is being prepared the legal representatives of the plaintiff (the injured person) will try to build a case based on both liabilities; this is termed the 'double barrelled action' and obviously increases the chance of success (although only one payment of compensation will be made if both liabilities are proved!).

LIABILITY AT COMMON LAW

Common law is a body of law that is contained within the reported decisions of courts. When arriving at a decision the judges will consider previous decisions in similar cases, the rule being that decisions of higher courts are binding on lower courts. If a situation comes before the court that does not fit the circumstances of previous decisions then the judge will make a decision that will further define and may extend or limit the law. The theory is that judges do not make law by this process but merely state what the law is.

The tort of negligence is that part of the common law that covers the many situations that may result in a person suffering injury or ill health. The legal concept of negligence is a vast subject and is constantly being refined and extended. Lord Macmillan said in a famous case (*Donoghue* v. *Stevenson*, 1932) that considered the duty of a manufacturer to those who may be injured by its products, that 'the categories of negligence are never closed'. Negligence or lack of care does not automatically give rise to a liability; it has to be shown that there was a legal duty to take care, that there has been a negligent breach of that duty and that damage has been suffered by the person to whom the duty was owed because of the breach of the duty.

The application of the tort of negligence to the employer–employee situation is a special division of this branch of the law. It has been established that it is the duty of an employer acting personally or through others to take reasonable care for the safety of his/her employees during their employment.

This duty is general but in particular has been held to include the following:

- the provision and maintenance of safe plant and machinery;
- a safe place of work and a safe means of access to the work and from it;
- competent fellow workers and supervision;
- a safe system of work.

Many cases reaching the courts deal with accidental injury or death rather than illness or disease and to most people the term 'safe' or 'safety' appears only to imply a situation where measures have been taken to prevent accidental injury. The common law has made it clear that the duty extends to taking care of workers' health as well (*Crookall* v. *Vickers-Armstrong*, 1955). Some of the duties defined by specific cases relating to health are outlined below.

An employer must consider the known disabilities of an individual worker when planning and setting up a safe system of work (*Paris* v. *Stepney Borough Council*, 1951). This case concerned a fitter with one eye who lost his other eye when hammering a rusty bolt. It was decided that his employers should have provided goggles for his use even though they would not normally provide them for workers with normal sight. This principle may be applied, for example, to those workers who have a history of lung problems who may be required to work in places where there is dust or fumes. However, further cases have shown that the employer is not liable if he or she does not know, or does not need to know, of the employee's disability, and that there is not normally a duty to carry out pre-employment medical examinations (unless there is a specific statutory requirement).

If, however, the employer is aware of a risk and sets a standard or level for exposure to it that is appropriate for safety then it is not considered negligent not to warn employees who may be specially sensitive to the risk if it is unlikely that the injury will occur. In a case concerning vibration white finger (*Joseph* v. *Ministry of Defence*, 1980) it was said that warning all the employees because there may be one exceptionally vulnerable one would cause unnecessary alarm. A sensitive employee could avoid this risk only by giving up the job.

There is a duty on the employer to enforce the safe system, not just to set it up. This duty, for example, would apply if an employer had decided that respirators were necessary to carry out a certain operation but did not put this system into operation or allowed it to lapse. It does not extend, however, to making sure that an experienced worker wears the respirator provided every time the opertion is carried out. The employer must take all reasonable measures to warn of the risks and precautions that are necessary (*General Cleaning Contractors* v. *Christmas*, 1953). Lord Justice Denning said that when an employer 'asks his men to work with dangerous substances, he must provide proper appliances to safeguard them, he must set in force the necessary system by which they use the appliances . . . and he must do his best to see that they adhere to it' (*Clifford* v. *Challen (Charles H.) & Son Ltd*, 1951).

If new techniques or plant are available somewhere in the world to deal with a particular risk then it is not negligent if an employer does not immediately use the new techniques. It may, however, be considered negligent not to introduce the measures if they are widely adopted in other similar companies and if the safety benefits are substantial. To decide what measures a reasonable employer should take the courts will consider what safety measures are currently available, then consider the disadvantages of these measures in terms of expense, effort, how far they will reduce the risk, interference with normal work, etc. against the seriousness of the risk. If the disadvantages of the measures outweigh the risk involved then it is not reasonable to expect the employer to provide the measures.

An employer is not negligent if he or she fails to take action against risks that were not known about at the time. In a 1969 case (*Tremain* v. *Pike*, 1969), there was no liability on an employer to take steps to protect workers against Weil's disease on a rat-infested farm as the risk was unknown. A similar case heard in 1988 (*Campbell* v. *Percy Bilton Ltd*, 1988) found in favour of a construction worker who contracted Weil's disease while working near a canal, the risk being well known by this date. Another case considered the claim for damages for the death of the wife of a shipyard worker from mesothelioma some time after 17 years of shaking out and washing her husband's dusty overalls (*Gunn* v. *Wallsend Slipway and Engineering Co. Ltd*, 1988). Her husband had been working with asbestos during this time and his legal representatives argued that at the time of his wife's exposure to the dusty overalls there was information that asbestos was harmful. However, the court decided that although information was available none of it applied to the risk of domestic exposure. No warnings in medical, industrial or official guidance literature were given at that time (pre-1965) that contact with the dust on clothes taken home could cause disease. The position is, of course, very different now.

LIABILITY FOR BREACH OF STATUTORY DUTY

Statutory duties are imposed on employers and others for the health and safety of employees and in some cases others. These statutory duties are enforced usually by penalties under the criminal system. The common law allows that where duties are imposed on an employer by a statute and a worker suffers an injury or disease due to failure by the employer to comply with the duty the worker can bring an action for damages. Sometimes this right of civil action is taken away by the statute, for example section 47 of the Health and Safety at Work etc. Act 1974 (regarding breaches of the general duties of employers and others contained in sections 2 to 8), and regulation 15 of the Management of Health and Safety at Work Regulations 1992, which states: 'Breach of a duty imposed by these Regulations shall not confer a right of action in any civil proceedings'.

To prove liability for breach of statutory duty it is not normally necessary to prove that the employer has been negligent; because of this it is said to be a **strict** or **absolute liability**. The worker must be able to prove that the following three factors applied:

- The statutory requirement imposed a duty on the employer that is intended to protect the worker against some injury or disease of a particular kind.
- The employer failed to carry out the duty.
- The breach of the duty resulted in the harm to the worker that the statute was introduced to prevent.

In cases of disease and illness the last factor may often be difficult to prove. Did the disease or illness actually result from the breach of the statutory duty? The principle followed by the courts is that if there has been exposure or increased exposure to work in conditions that may result in disease then that is considered sufficient evidence (*Bonnington Castings Ltd* v. *Wardlaw*, 1956). The employee must in all cases prove his or her case by the ordinary standard of proof in civil actions: 'He must make it appear at least on the balance of probabilities the breach of duty caused or materially contributed to his injury'. The case concerned a worker who contracted silicosis; the statutory requirement related to extraction equipment but the worker was exposed to other dusts as well as to those that would have been extracted. His case succeeded as the court accepted that the breach of the requirement resulted in increased exposure.

Statutory requirements may be absolute or qualified by words such as 'so far as is practicable' or 'reasonably practicable'. Examples of these are given below.

The Asbestos (Prohibitions) Regulations 1985, regulation 7, 'No person shall install asbestos insulation' is an obvious example of an absolute requirement.

The Control of Substances Hazardous to Health Regulations 1988 (COSHH), regulation 9(1), states: 'Every employer who provides any control measure to meet the requirements of regulation 7 shall ensure that it is maintained in an efficient state, in efficient working order and in good repair'. This type of phrase relating to maintenance is repeated in many regulations and has been held to be an absolute requirement in that it describes a result to be achieved rather than the means of achieving it.

The Control of Lead at Work Regulations 1988, regulation 14, is similar to the COSHH requirement above but introduces the word 'practicable'. 'Every employer who provides any control measure, respiratory protective equipment, protective clothing or other thing or facility . . . shall ensure, so far as is practicable, that it is maintained in an efficient state, in efficient working order and in good repair.' The word 'practicable' has been held to mean possible in the light of current knowledge and invention and does not include considerations such as cost or inconvenience (*Adsett* v. *K and L Steelfounders and Engineers Ltd*, 1953).

The Control of Asbestos at Work Regulations 1987, regulation 12, state: 'Every employer shall prevent or where this is not reasonably practicable, reduce to the lowest level reasonably practicable, the spread of asbestos from any place where work with asbestos is carried out'. The term 'reasonably practicable' is used in many statutory duties and has been held to imply that a judgement must be made by the employer about the seriousness of the risk on the one hand against the sacrifice in terms of cost, time and trouble of the necessary measures to deal with the risk on the other. If the risk is insignificant compared with the sacrifice then it is not reasonably practicable for the employer to provide the measures (*Edwards* v. *National Coal Board*, 1949). This judgement must be made before the risk is faced by the worker and the size and financial standing of the employer does not affect the calculation – if it is reasonably practicable for a large organization to provide the measures the same applies to a small organization – the important factor is the level of risk.

This 'reasonably practicable' test can be considered to be the basis of **risk assessment**, which is now an explicit requirement of most new legis-lation and therefore it is argued that employers should find little difficulty in complying with the new legislation, since to comply with the previous requirements, in particular the general duties of the Health and Safety at Work etc. Act 1974, there was an implied requirement of risk assessment to provide measures that were 'reasonably practicable'.

The 'reasonably practicable' principle has been the cause of some problems with the introduction of European directives, which are written in strict liability terms, into UK legislation. The UK courts interpret statutory requirements strictly and if an absolute requirement will prevent some equipment or process continuing then that is not the concern of the courts. Some European countries' legal systems allow for a consideration of reasonableness in the final decision of a court.

Many regulations require the employer to provide some form of personal protective equipment, for example regulation 7(3) of COSHH requires the employer, in situations where the control measures he or she has provided do not prevent or adequately control exposure to substances hazardous to health, to '. . . provide those employees with personal protective equipment as will adequately control their exposure to substances hazardous to health'. This requirements is written into many other regulations and it has been held that the duty is not complied with if the employer merely makes the equipment available on request; it is the duty of the employer to give the equipment to the employee, perhaps even putting the equipment in to his or her hands (*Crouch* v. *British Rail Engineering Ltd*, 1989). Some form of record keeping is therefore essential if employers want to be able to prove that they have provided the proper equipment.

As indicated in the brief outline above the subject is extremely complicated and can lead to unsatisfactory results for the disabled worker. The need to prove negligence or breach of statutory duty will inevitably mean that some workers who have suffered disease or ill health will fail to obtain compensation and yet their condition may be as serious or worse than that of those who succeed. The cost of the system is staggering – the Royal Commission on Civil Liability and Compensation for Personal Injury under the chairmanship of Lord Pearson (Royal Commission on Civil Liability and Compensation for Personal Injury, 1978) calculated that it cost 87 pence for every £1 paid to plaintiffs by the tort system.

EMPLOYERS' LIABILITY INSURANCE

The most important form of insurance relating to the payment of damages to workers who suffer ill health from their work is employers' liability insurance. Employers in almost every country will need insurance to meet this liability in some form or other, unless they are big enough to take on the financial risk themselves. It is a legal requirement in the UK under the Employers' Liability (Compulsory Insurance) Act 1969. The Act came into force on 1st January 1972 and requires all employers (other than certain exempt employers such as government bodies) to obtain insurance cover from an authorized insurer. The insurance policy will provide compensation to an employee if there is legal liability in the event of death, injury or disease that is caused during the period of insurance and arises out of and in the course of this employment. The insurers will also meet legal costs and expenses in dealing with the claim.

It must be emphasized again that the insurance will not provide payment for injury or illness where there is no legal liability. Evidence of negligence and/or breach of statutory duty as outlined above will be required before any payment is made. This does not mean, however, that insurers wait for the outcome of a case in the courts to pay compensation. It is estimated that over 90% of all claims are settled without going to court and of the cases set down for trial only about 25% actually receive a full hearing. The pressure to settle is very powerful when the enormous legal costs, medical reports, expert witness costs, expenses, etc. of going to court are taken into account.

The disease must be contracted or caused during the period of insurance. This leads to obvious difficulties in the case of diseases such as cancers or chronic lung disease where the exposure may have been 15 or 20 years before, the symptoms of the disease appearing long after exposure. It is likely that the insurers will have changed over the years, but the insurer at the time of the cause will still be required to pay if liability can be proved. This is termed a 'long tail liability' by insurers. In the case of a developing disease such as asbestosis or deafness, all insurers involved with an employer over the period of exposure may agree to pay a proportion of the compensation related to the time that their policy was in force.

A claim for disease is received by an employer, the employee, or past employee, claiming that it was caused by exposure to some condition many years ago. The employer may find that he or she is unable to track down the insurers of that time and the employer is therefore, liable to meet the cost of the claim him or herself. To meet this eventuality it may be possible for an employer to arrange with his present insurers to provide extended cover under a current policy to include all claims made during the period of the policy – not all insurers are prepared to take on this sort of risk, however.

The policy will specify the type of business that it covers and also will list exclusions that it does not cover. Premium rates are calculated on the basis of the type of risk, size of organization, previous claims record, etc. Problems can arise if a business expands into other areas of activity that are not covered by its policy such as a construction company deciding to set up an asbestos stripping operation without informing its insurers and obtaining their agreement. Other situations may lead to unintentional loss of cover such as acquisitions or mergers of companies whose activities are outside the scope of the parent company. Cover may also be limited geographically and will usually cover employees working overseas only on a temporary basis and will normally exclude any work in the United States.

The Employers' Liability (Compulsory Insurance) Act sets a minimum indemnity of £2 million for any one occurrence; however, most insurers have traditionally provided unlimited cover for this form of insurance. This position appears to be changing and the insurance world has warned that in future the minimum cover of £2 million may only be offered with options to purchase increased cover by paying a higher premium. This is due to the difficulties experienced in obtaining reinsurance in the market (the process of spreading the financial risk between several insurers) as well as to an awareness of the catastrophes of recent times such as the Piper Alpha disaster. There have been a number of individual settlements well in excess of £1 million. There is also a move to structured settlements; this form of settlement for the very large award provides a lump sum, part of which is in the form of an annuity which provides an income for life.

Another development in the last 10 years or so is 'forum shopping'. This is the attempt to get your case heard in the country and court that is likely to provide the highest possible payment. In most cases this involves trying to prove some link with the United States – that the employee was injured there, the product that caused the injury was manufactured there or that one of the defendants is based in the United States. Awards made in the United States are about 10 times larger than those for similar cases in the UK. This approach was used in the case of claims on behalf of victims of the Piper Alpha disaster and has been used after some UK air crashes. The approach sometimes results in what is termed a 'Mid-Atlantic settlement' where the compensation offered is less than an US court might have awarded but substantially more than would have been likely from a UK or other European court.

In the past, claims for disease have been a small proportion of employers' liability claims. The Pearson Commission (Cane, 1993) reported that in 1973 there were 114 700 claims for injury (90 500 payments) and only 2900 claims for disease (1700 payments). More recent statistics split this way are not readily available but total successful claims from 1988 to 1991 varied between 110 000 and over 140 000 (Association of British Insurers, annual). The proportion of injury claims to disease claims is changing according to a representative of an insurance company who stated in 1993 that between 1986 and 1990 the number of accident claims rose by 45% but claims for disease rose by 90% over the same period.

As is implied from the above figures only a small number of workers actually claim compensation. The Pearson Commission (Cane, 1993) estimated that only about 10.5% of those who suffer injuries or disease at work obtained compensation through the tort system. Several reasons have been suggested for this reluctance of workers to claim, although evidence is strong that workers are becoming less reluctant.

Medical knowledge of the causes of disease and advanced methods of diagnosis are improving all the time and making it easier for a worker to prove a claim. The trade unions are particularly active in pursuing claims for disease on behalf of their members.

Claims consciousness is increasing. That is the knowledge that a worker can make a claim for his or her disability or disease. Part of the reason for this is the removal of the prohibition on solicitors to advertise. It is now common to see advertisements in newspapers and hear them on local radio inviting those who have been injured or suffered illness at work to have a free interview to discuss the possibility of a claim. Claims consciousness in the United States is very high; it is claimed that any American injured in a road accident will call for his lawyer, doctor and priest – in that order!

There is a move to allowing 'no win, no fee' agreements between lawyers and clients in the UK such as are common in other countries – the contingent fee system. This arrangement has been arrived at partly to deal with the changes in the Legal Aid scheme which have dramatically reduced the numbers eligible for legal aid. With the 'no win, no fee' system the claimant will not have to pay legal fees if he or she loses the action, but there is the disadvantage that he or she will have to pay the opponents' substantial costs.

Another proposal in the UK is that employers should face punitive damages similar to the damages that apply in countries such as the United States of America and Australia (The Law Commission). The tort system aims to make full compensation for a claim in order to put the plaintiff back in the position he or she would have been in if the accident or disease had not occurred. The cost includes loss of income, loss of benefits, costs of ongoing medical care, adaptations to living accommodation, etc. Punitive damages, as their name suggests, go further than trying to provide full restitution to the injured person; they are intended to act as a form of deterrent and provide an example of the seriousness with which the law treats those who fail to consider the health and safety of their employees. A counter argument to this approach is that this is precisely what the criminal justice system is designed to do.

The cost of insurance has risen dramatically in recent years. This is related to increases in numbers and sizes of claims. Over the same period industrial activity has been affected by the recession and the numbers of people in work have fallen. Many companies have had annual increases in their premiums of between 30% and 40% and some insurers are warning that increases of between 75% and 100% may be required in the future. Combined premiums for employers' liability and public liability rose from £966 million in 1988 to £1216 million in 1991 (Association of British Insurers, annual).

The 1990 Labour Force Survey, carried out for the UK Health and

Safety Executive in 1989/90 (Hodgson *et al.*, 1993), found that nearly 6% of adults believed they had suffered a work related illness in the period covered. Of the diseases reported, 40% were musculo-skeletal (593 000 estimate); others included deafness, chronic poisoning, stress, skin conditions, etc. These figures are far greater than the figures for accidental injury over the same period (injury figures obtained from the survey suggest that only about 30% of accidents required to be reported to the Health and Safety Executive by the Reporting of Injuries, Diseases and Dangerous Occurrences Regulations 1985 are in fact reported).

The insurers are becoming increasingly concerned at the growing number of possible areas for claims in the future. An out of court settlement for £15 000 to a woman who became chronically ill as a result, she claimed, of working in an office where a number of colleagues smoked is likely to lead to many similar claims for passive smoking related illness. Despite recent controversial statements by a judge that repetitive strain injury (RSI) does not exist, it is clear that there are going to be growing numbers of claims for various work related upper limb disorders from keyboard operators, production line workers, etc. Another area anxiously being studied is that of worker stress. The Labour Force Survey referred to above indicated that many people are suffering from stress or depression as a result of their work. Of the workers who claimed to have suffered a work related illness in the period studied, 8.2% said it was due to stress. Teachers in particular reported a high level of stress-related illness – 46% of all teachers claiming to have suffered illness due to their work claim it was due to stress.

Some insurers are becoming more proactive in their role in an effort to reduce claims. Traditionally insurers set premiums by reference to risk tables for various activities or industries, numbers of employees, number of claims in the previous five years, etc. It is becoming increasingly common for insurers, brokers and even underwriters to visit an employer's premises to check on conditions before renewing a policy, particularly if there has been a significant number of claims. Some employers have found themselves being turned down for renewal because of their claims record and are finding that other insurers will not take them on. As employers' liability insurance is a legal requirement this can effectively put them out of business. In these cases the employer will need to convince the insurers that health and safety will, in future, be properly managed; in particular any health hazard that may lead to future claims for chronic illness must be fully controlled to current standards. Probably one of the first actions recommended to an employer in this situation would be to obtain the services of a specialist consultant.

STATE INSURANCE SYSTEMS

In addition to the tort system outlined above there is a state insurance scheme designed to provide some form of compensation to workers. Unlike the tort system there is no need to prove negligence and the scheme does not set out to provide full compensation to the worker but is usually based on some set scale of payments.

In the UK as far as diseases are concerned the Social Security Act provides benefit if a disease has been prescribed by the Social Security (Industrial Injuries) (Prescribed Diseases) Regulations. A disease may be prescribed if

- it ought to be treated, having regard to its causes and incidence and other relevant considerations, as a risk of occupation and not as a risk common to all persons; and
- it is such that, in the absence of special circumstances, the attribution of particular cases to the nature of the employment can be established with reasonable certainty.

Because of difficulties in meeting the above criteria many diseases are not prescribed and therefore fall outside the scope of the system.

To make a claim under this system the worker must be suffering the particular prescribed disease, in some cases to the extent defined, and be able to show that he or she is or was employed in a specific process or type of work. Note that only employees are covered by this scheme. A proposal by the Industrial Injuries Advisory Council that self-employed workers be included in the scheme was rejected by the UK government in 1993 on the grounds that they are expected to make their own insurance arrangements. There were estimated to be 3.3 million self-employed workers in 1991. The UK scheme is financed by taxation and by flat rate contributions paid mainly by the employer and partly by the employee.

Almost every country now has some form of workers' compensation scheme. This form of compensation is the oldest form of social security with the introduction of a law in Germany in 1884. There has been a trend in recent times to bring occupational injury schemes into line with other social security. This removes the problem of identifying whether a particular injury or disease was caused by work. Switzerland has covered all accidental injury in the same way since 1911 and New Zealand has had a no fault system since 1974 that includes ill health from occupational causes. Australia did prepare a scheme which compensated for all accidents and disease but a change of government led to the scheme being shelved. The Netherlands is the only country that pays disability benefit regardless of cause.

The occupational schemes are operated in a variety of ways with a variety of benefits and methods of funding. All occupational schemes include occupational disease (with the problems this entails as outlined above of establishing causation). Following the German lead in 1925, many occupational schemes include travel to and from work (not the UK).

Benefits normally include the following: medical expenses in countries where there is no national health provision; short-term incapacity benefit for time off work, which ranges in different countries from 50–100% of normal wage, sometimes payable after a waiting period; permanent incapacity benefit for those who will not be able to work again, normally in the form of a pension. A further benefit in countries such as Austria, France, Germany, Ireland, Israel, The Netherlands and Switzerland is arrangements for retraining and in some cases guaranteed employment.

The cost of administering the UK social security scheme was estimated by the Pearson Commission as 11 pence for every £1 paid to claimants; the New Zealand Accident Scheme amounted to 8% of the benefits paid. This can be compared with the costs of the tort system, which was estimated as 87 pence for every £1 as noted above. The tort system, however, aims to provide full compensation to those who can establish negligence whereas the other systems aim to compensate everyone who is injured regardless of fault. Very few people receive compensation under the tort system, however, and as it is so expensive to administer there must eventually be pressure to produce a more cost-effective and fairer system for those who suffer injury or disease from whatever cause. This is, of course, a political matter. Anyone who wishes to read further on this topic is referred to the Pearson Commission Report, and other publications may be of interest (Cane, 1993).

CONSULTANTS AND LIABILITY

People who offer professional advice and services such as engineers, architects, doctors, accountants, safety consultants, etc. are subject to claims being made against them in the event of some loss, injury or damage which can be shown to be due to any neglect, error or omission made by them in the course of their business.

A typical clause from a professional indemnity policy would say something along these lines: 'Insurers agree to indemnify the Insured, in respect of loss arising from any claim or claims for breach of duty which may be made against them and reported to the insured during the currency of this policy by reason of any neglect, error or omission whenever or whatever committed or alleged to have been committed in the conduct of the Insured's business in the professional capacity as stated in the schedule by the Insured on or by any person now or who may have been heretofore or may hereafter be in the employment of the Insured.'

The courts in considering the liability of those who are professionals expect a high standard of care. The test in establishing whether an occupational health consultant has been negligent is whether he or she has carried out the task with the degree of skill appropriate to a reasonably competent member of the profession. The consultant therefore may be negligent even though he or she carries out the task to the best of his or her ability.

The consultant may end up having to pay the whole of the damages to the injured employee of the client by whom the consultant was engaged. In the case of a construction site accident where a worker was injured by material falling from a hoist, the employer had not complied with the statutory requirements relating to hoists and the safety consultant inspecting the site was held not to have sufficiently emphasized the importance of defects. The damages were awarded against both the employer and the consultant, each being liable for a proportion. The employer then successfully argued that he had relied on the consultant's advice and therefore the consultant should also pay the employer's proportion. The consultant was required to pay the whole amount (*Driver* v. *William Willet (Contractors) Ltd and others*, 1969).

In the Abbeystead disaster a massive methane gas explosion occurred in a water pumping station while members of the public were being shown around. This resulted in claims being made against the water authority that owned the pumping station, the contractor that built the structure and the consultant engineering practice that designed it. Damages in the High Court were awarded against all three organizations but the final decision in the Court of Appeal was that the consultant engineers had to meet all claims.

As noted in the typical clause above, the policy will indemnify the consultant for matters concerning the consultant's business in the particular professional capacity that will be set out in the schedule of the policy. In other words an occupational health consultant will be indemnified for claims arising out of advice and services he or she may provide on occupational health matters but may not be indemnified if he or she gives advice on environmental matters (that is pollution of air, water or land), major pollution takes place and some important omission or error was made by the consultant. This is not an academic point – warnings have been issued by insurers regarding this as the costs involved in pollution can be enormous. It is very easy for health and safety consultants to stray into giving advice on environmental matters as the disciplines are so similar, but unless cover is provided it could prove to be extremely expensive.

Some practical points for individual occupational health consultants to bear in mind are outlined below. Larger consultancy partnerships, companies, laboratories, etc. will probably have covered these matters in the systems they have developed for quality assurance, particularly if they have achieved accreditation under some scheme such as ISO 9000/BS 5750 or NAMAS.

Obtain professional indemnity insurance with a suitable level of cover and make sure that your insurer is aware of the full scope of your activities; particularly important is the possibility of carrying out work in other countries.

Make clear to your clients the purpose, nature and extent of work you have carried out in any reports and correspondence. There is a big difference between a simple 'walk through survey' and a thorough occupational health survey involving observations of working practices, measurement of concentrations of dusts or fumes, checking ventilation flow rates, and so on; this difference may not be apparent many years later when a claim is made. The limits in terms of time on site, ability to make detailed examinations, etc. must be clearly stated and recorded for future reference.

Record all advice given including telephone advice. Claims, particularly for disease, may come years after your contact with a client and memories will fade, people will deny what you said or will be untraceable.

Keep a diary and record visits, inspections, telephone calls, receipt of letters, sending reports, taking samples, etc. It is an amazing memory jogger, even many years later, of things done and said and may prove invaluable in the event of a claim.

Keep records of your work. Notebooks, *not* scraps of paper, should be used for notes made on site, records of discussions, measurements, names of people met on site and so on, and these should be kept with all copies of reports, letters and other documents relating to a client. Note that the time limit for making a claim for disease is three years after the date that the person has knowledge of the condition. Therefore to cater for diseases which take a long time to show any symptoms it would appear wise not to discard any records at all.

Make sure that you keep up to date with current developments in your professional discipline. The standard to be applied is that of a reasonably competent fellow professional. Information that was readily available at the time that you carried out your work is likely to be produced as evidence in a claim. It is particularly important to have a thorough understanding of current official guidance and recommendations such as Health and Safety Executive literature and, of course, statutory requirements and Approved Codes of Practice. Ensure you have access to the latest versions of important documents such as

HSE's *EH 40 Occupational Exposure Limits* (HSE, annual). It may be useful to explore the possibility of subscribing to some form of information service, university library or database if you do not have ready access in your own organization to information.

If a particular project is outside your field of expertise you may be better off turning down the work despite the attractive possibility of high fees or long-term work. It is, however, common for a consultant to carry out work in very different areas; for example, a consultant may be asked to carry out an occupational health survey in a printing works when previous experience is in general manufacturing. By the application of sound basic principles and some research he or she may feel able to accept the work. If you take on work that is not in your normal line of business, make sure that you are not outside the terms of your insurance and that you research any particular industry or specific process guidelines.

In conclusion, as a consultant you put your head on the block. Carry out your work in a conscientious manner but make sure that you are covered if things go wrong. The courts try to bend over backwards to give compensation to injured workers and the more expert a person claims to be the more likely it is that the court will attach liability to him or her if there is evidence of negligence.

REFERENCES

Adsett v. *K and L Steelfounders and Engineers Ltd* [1953] 1 *All England Law Reports* 97; 1 *Weekly Law Reports* 773.

Association of British Insurers (annual) *Statistics of Association of British Insurers,* 51 Gresham Street, London, EC2V 7HQ.

Bonnington Castings Ltd v. *Wardlaw* [1956] *Appeal Case* 613; 1 *All England Law Reports* 615; 2 *Weekly Law Reports* 707.

Campbell v. *Percy Bilton Ltd* (1988) Unreported Case.

Cane, P. (1993) *Atiyah's Accidents, Compensation and the Law* (Law in Context Series), Butterworths, London, UK.

Clifford v. *Challen (Charles H) & Son Ltd* [1951] 1 *All England Law Reports* 72; [1951] 1 *King's Bench (Law Reports)* 495.

Crookall v. *Vickers-Armstrong Ltd* [1955] 2 *All England Law Reports* 12; *Law Times* 198.

Crouch v. *British Rail Engineering Ltd* [1989] *Appeal Case.*

Donoghue v. *Stevenson* [1932] *Appeal Case* 562 reference in *Munkman's Employers' Liability at Common Law,* Butterworths, UK.

Driver v. *William Willet (Contractors) Ltd* and others [1969] 1 *All England Law Reports* 665.

Edwards v. *National Coal Board* [1949] 1 *King's Bench (Law Reports)* 704; 1 *All England Law Reports,* 9 April, 743.

General Cleaning Contractors v. *Christmas* [1953] *Appeal Case* 180; [1952] 2 *All England Law Reports* 1110.

Gunn v. *Wallsend Slipway and Engineering Co. Ltd* (1988) Unreported case.

HSE (annual) *EH40 Occupational Exposure Limits*, HSE, Sudbury, UK.

Hodgson, J.T., Jones, J.R., Elliott, R.C. and Osman, J. (1993) Self-reported work-related illness. *Health and Safety Executive Research Paper 33*, HSE Books, Sudbury, UK.

Joseph v. *Ministry of Defence* (1980) *Times Law Reports*, 4 March.

Munkman, J. (1990) *Munkman's Employer's Liability at Common Law*, Butterworths, London, UK.

Paris v. *Stepney Borough Council* [1951] *Appeal Case* 367; 1 *All England Law Reports* 42; *Times Law Reports*, 5 Jan. 1951; *Law Journal*, 29 Dec. 1950, 100 (4431), 719.

The Law Commission Consultative Paper No. 132. Aggravated, exemplary and restitutionary damages.

Royal Commission on Civil Liability and Compensation for Personal Injury (1978) *Report*, HMSO, London.

Tremain v. *Pike* [1969] 3 *All England Law Reports* 1303.

PART TWO

Rehabilitation for work

4

Jean Raper

INTRODUCTION

'Rehabilitation for work is nothing new, it's been going on for years. Someone is off long term sick, he comes back and we carry him for a bit then he does his own job.' That form of rehabilitation has gone on for years and, in many cases, has proved successful. However, in many cases it has not. There are no statistics available to demonstrate the outcomes of this form of rehabilitation for work, it is fraught with risk of litigation against the employer if not successful, and also places a burden on the co-workers who do the 'carrying'. Generally, however, the long-term sick employee stays away from work either until his or her general practitioner signs him or her fit to return or he or she is dismissed on the grounds of health status.

When we consider the cost of employing someone, the cost of training him or her to perform whatever task, the cost of overtime when he or she is away and the cost of recruiting and training someone else if he or she doesn't come back, a more formal approach to rehabilitation for work becomes very attractive. Add to the above the cost of liability claims against the employer for both occupational ill health and industrial injury and a programme which involves obvious cost limitation benefits becomes a necessity.

In 1991 UK insurers (excluding Lloyd's) paid out £583 million in employers' liability insurance claims. Uninsured losses are estimated to cost around £4–6 billion and 'when account is taken of the hidden costs borne by the public (e.g. National Health Service) and the victim, we are approaching figures (£10–15 billion per annum) which amount to circa 2% of the gross national product' (Ballard, 1994a).

There are obviously many areas of occupational health practice which can be effectively used to help reduce this tremendous cost to employers, individuals and society generally. Rehabilitation for work is one of those areas.

ABSENCE CONTROL

A starting point for any employer wishing to address the issues around rehabilitation for work has to be a well understood absence control procedure. Such a procedure will require commitment from all levels of employees and will contain clear lines of responsibility for reporting and monitoring absence. It should also make evident the fact that

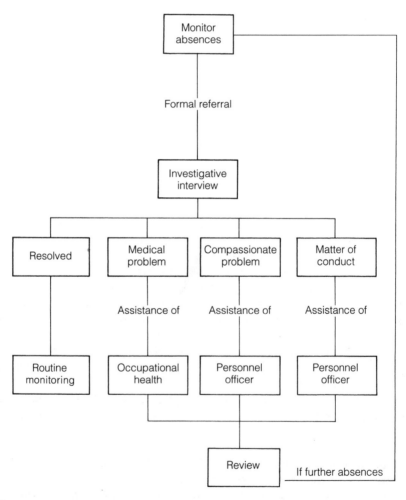

Figure 4.1   An example of an absence control procedure.

absence control starts at recruitment and continues throughout employment. An example procedure is given in Figure 4.1.

Absence control is not only a disciplinary tool for managers; success which can be measured in positive outcomes will only be achieved if the procedure leads to proactive as well as reactive intervention. It should provide a method of investigating absence and its causes. Short and medium-term absence will need to be reviewed regularly while longer term absence will present the manager with a different set of problems. To enable consistency in the methods of dealing with absence it is recommended that a standard measure be introduced for each type of absence. The measures for frequent short-term absence should include, at some point, a health assessment to ensure there is no underlying unidentified medical cause. However, there is rarely a need to consider occupational health involvement in rehabilitation of such employees.

Intermediate and long-term absences present a different problem. Many managers will need assurances that their employees are fit for the work they have to do and that their health will not be further challenged by returning to such work. For occupational health advice to be of value it is essential that early referral is made. In a report on the management of sickness absence in Local Authorities (Audit Commission, 1990) it was noted that '. . . the point at which those on long-term sickness are referred to the occupational health unit varied from five weeks to six months. Lengthy delays then occur . . .' The report went on to detail the benefits of early referral and the potential to arrange an early return to work. It is obviously in everyone's interest for decisions on the employee's health status and future employment potential to be made as soon as possible.

Therefore the elements of absence control that most affect rehabilitation for work are early intervention and early referral by managers. There are, however, other elements of general management that are equally important. Under regulation 8 of the Management of Health and Safety at Work Regulations 1992, a duty is placed on the employer to 'provide his employees with comprehensive and relevant information on (a) the risks to their health and safety . . .' (HSC, 1992). This outcome of 'risk assessment' has the potential to have a major impact on decisions relevant to rehabilitation for work, e.g. where the risks identified could have a direct or indirect effect on the employee's ability to maintain him or herself in health. Such an 'assessment' is, therefore, an essential part of the information a manager should provide when referring employees for occupational health advice and should be attached to the referral document which should detail management intervention and current knowledge of the employee's health status. Other useful information will include copies of the employee's attendance records, job description and/or job specification together with any relevant training records, thus providing the occupational health professional with a broad base of information on which to make any recommendations.

The following absence control policy is included for guidance on the setting of standard measures and their implementation.

ABSENCE CONTROL POLICY

1. Commitment

'......' recognizes that the commitment and responsibility for controlling absence should be manifest at all levels of the Company.

2. Responsibilities

The monitoring and control of absence on a day to day basis will rest with section heads and/or supervisors. In order to ensure that section heads or supervisors are managing the situation adequately line managers must take responsibility for overseeing their performance. This method of control will lead to problems being addressed before they get out of hand and to appropriate support being made available when and where it is needed.

3. Information

Accurate, readily available and clearly understood information is an essential adjunct to effective absence control. The control of absence by section heads/supervisors and line managers is difficult without the appropriate information. Setting targets to reduce absence will be of little value if monitoring information is not available for performance comparison.

It is recognized that different types of information are needed at different levels in the organization. The use of clearly presented information will not only be helpful to managers seeking to identify key problems but can also be used to demonstrate to employees how absence levels in their Section/Department compare with Departmental/Company averages.

4. Training

The key role of section heads/supervisors and line managers in controlling absence has already been mentioned. It is important that they acquire the skills, support and guidance they need to carry out this role successfully. Guidance outlining the agreed procedures will be made available.

5. Processes

The processes for controlling absence fall into various categories: recruitment, monitoring and follow-up action.

6. Recruitment

Guidance for potential employees, giving advice on health challenges associated with those jobs known to present some risk, is to be issued with job application forms. The guidance is designed to give an applicant the opportunity to make an informed decision before applying for such jobs. Recruiters will need to take cognisance of this guidance.

Health Declarations will be completed by all potential employees prior to appointment. This information will be treated as strictly confidential and will be available only to Occupational Health staff.

Factual information related to an applicant's previous attendance and time-keeping should be sought from referees. Where possible cause for concern is identified, enquiry into the background to the poor attendance is advised.

Induction should be used as a means of developing positive attitudes to good attendance. It should also be used to familiarize new employees with the requirements for reporting absence. This practice need not be time-consuming and could be incorporated into a line manager's initial meetings with an employee.

7. Reporting absences

Procedures for reporting absences should be clear and well publicized. All staff should be issued with a personal copy of the reporting requirements. The reporting requirements should make it clear who should report absence, how, to whom, when and the information that should be provided. Precise requirements for reporting sickness absence help emphasize the importance of good attendance.

8. Short-term absence

The reason for a short-term absence, i.e. one to three (or more) days, should be established by the section head/supervisor.

The corporate standard measure for formal intervention in the case of short-term absences will be any two periods of absence in any three months. If there are concerns about an individual's pattern of absence then formal intervention should be made without waiting for the corporate standard measure to trigger such intervention.

Dependent upon the findings there may be a need to consider earlier intervention. Section heads/supervisors should seek advice from the Personnel Officer or Occupational Health Nurse (Figure 4.1).

9. Sickness absence—self and medically certified

The corporate standard measure for dealing with this category will relate to absences of four days to five weeks. Section heads/ supervisors will carry out 'return to work' interviews with all employees following this type of absence. The purpose of these interviews will be not only to ensure that employees know that their absences are noted and taken seriously but also to provide an opportunity to identify any underlying problems. Where the need for intervention is identified advice should be sought from the Personnel Officer or Occupational Health Nurse on any appropriate action. Any four such absences in a 12-month period must be referred to Occupational Health.

10. Long-term sickness absence

All cases of long-term sickness absence will be referred to the Occupational Health Nurse at six weeks. This will form the corporate standard measure.

ASSESSMENT

Employment assessment must be an essential element of any rehabilitation for work programme. Such assessment is available through the Department of Employment's Employment Service which has responsibility for arranging such services through its Placement, Assessment and Counselling Teams (PACTs). There are also organizations which advise on assessment for specific disabilities (Hawkes and Paschkes Bell, 1993). There are, of course, many private consultants providing similar services.

However, many occupational health professionals, working in coordination with their employer's personnel and training officers, will be able to create their own assessment process. Some personnel and training officers will have qualifications in the use of various assessment tests and questionnaires and will have formal links with occupational psychologists. Where this type of facility is available there will rarely be a need to involve PACTs in the management of those needing short-term rehabilitation. In a paper presented at the International Commission on Occupational Health Congress 1993, it was clearly demonstrated that intensive, combined intervention with a group of workers suffering from neck and shoulder pain did produce a marked reduction in absenteeism when compared with a control group (Nygren *et al.*, 1993). Many other presenters were able to demonstrate the value of co-working, not only between health care workers but also between workers, managers, trainers, etc. The benefits of an 'in-house' assessment process are obvious. In most cases both those conducting the assessment and those being assessed know the processes and organization of the employer and are aware of the potential for job redesign, retraining or redeployment should any or all of these elements be necessary.

The occupational health nurse or doctor will provide assessment of health and fitness ability and will be able to comment on any restrictions these elements of capability will place on the employee. They will also be able to advise on the likely length of time the employee will require to become fully rehabilitated. In the Department of Social Security's consultation document on the medical assessment for Incapacity Benefit (issued 1st December, 1993) proposals were put forward for a new system for the assessment of medical incapacity for work. The tests are designed to assess an individual's ability to carry out a range of work-related activities rather than his or her ability to do specific jobs. The criteria eventually agreed will obviously be of value to occupational health professionals as assessment tools and will link more closely to the criteria for various benefits, and thus financial support, for the rehabilitation for work of employees.

Assessment is, however, a double-edged sword and may well lead to advice that the employee is not capable of achieving rehabilitation for any type of work within the company. In these few, but nevertheless unfortunate, cases properly formulated support programmes should be offered. These programmes, which may already be available as part of employee retirement or redundancy services, should include advice from the occupational health professional on related health issues.

DISABILITY LEAVE

Disability leave is a relatively new concept that has been formally presented by the Royal National Institute for the Blind (Hawkes and Paschkes Bell, 1993) following a feasibility study into future provision of rehabilitation services (Paschkes Bell and Wavell, 1990). Though the study related to the rehabilitation needs of the blind, it was obvious that the same criteria should apply to people across a range of disability. The concept of disability leave was devised to help those who become disabled while in employment, so they could avoid having to give up their jobs unnecessarily and to help employers retain the skills and experience of their employees.

The project is mainly aimed at those who become newly disabled or whose disability progressively deteriorates. It is designed to facilitate informed decision making by both the employer and employee. Short-term disability following accident or ill health challenges is not commented on, and seems less well understood. There is no statutory provision for the 'returner' and this frequently means that workers remain off sick for excessively long periods of time. They lose contact with co-workers and become isolated and deskilled. In some cases they lose their employment.

While the RNIB project is aimed at those whose disability will have long-term implications for them, many of the concepts apply equally to those whose rehabilitation needs will be shorter term and more easily resolved. An interesting element of the project is the recognition that '. . . this may sometimes mean that Sickness Leave and Disability Leave will overlap. This means that the employee may continue to receive any financial help he or she is entitled to under Sickness Leave while undertaking an employment assessment and any further training that may be required'. The protection this would offer a returner would make the implementation of a rehabilitation programme more acceptable to managers and worker representatives, and would facilitate retraining for redeployees.

All the elements of the project could apply equally to those needing long or short-term support for rehabilitation and thus provide useful guidance for occupational health professionals wishing to introduce a Rehabilitation for Work programme to their employer.

DISABILITY

Disability can be broadly defined to mean a physical, sensory or mental impairment that substantially limits one or more of life's activities. Disablement for work means that the person defined as disabled is prevented from carrying out all the functions of his or her post. A disabled person is not necessarily ill, though like all other employees they may become ill and it may well be that the illness will be exacerbated by, or indeed exacerbate, the disability.

In the 1991 UK census it was revealed that some 14% of the population experienced some form of disabling impairment.

Disability, therefore, is a normal part of life for many people. They may have worked in a full capacity for years and quite suddenly find that, because of deterioration in their condition or change in work process or some other challenge, they are no longer able to function fully in their job. Others who have suffered or are suffering from ill health problems may well go on to become permanently disabled. Acquiring a disability or experiencing gradual loss of function can lead to loss of confidence, and may, unless proper advice is available, lead to an employee making ill-considered decisions about termination of employment. It is important to recognize that this is bound to be much more of a problem for the person concerned than for the employer or his or her adviser.

Retention of disabled employees is an important strategy for any employer. Many readers will be aware of the Disabled Persons (Employment) Acts 1944 and 1958. The 1944 Act as amended by the 1958 Act established a voluntary register of disabled people. Under these Acts an employer of 20 or more workers is required to employ a quota of registered disabled people. The standard quota is 3% of an employer's total workforce though it is not an offence to be below this quota. The Act is generally interpreted in terms of recruitment but it is little use having positive action strategies in recruitment if disabled people are leaving the organization at the same rate that they are being recruited. Recognizing this the 1994 Act includes section 9, paragraph 5:

> An employer must not discharge a registered disabled person without 'reasonable cause' if he is below his quota or if discharge would bring him below it.

An employer, therefore, should make every effort to retain any disabled employee, thus adhering to the spirit of the law, especially when it is as clear as this one. A disabled person, because of the 'stigma' perceived to be attached to registration, may choose not to apply for such registration. It is important to recognize the anxieties of such employees and not to place unnecessary pressure on them merely to achieve quotas. In the main it is the responsibility of the personnel function to provide the lead advice on matters related to employment; however, in the case of retention of those with an existing but deteriorating disability, or those who have become disabled whilst in employment, there are other professional services that can provide specific help.

It is likely that all occupational health professionals will have had contact at one time or another with the Disablement Advisory Service (DAS), Disablement Resettlement Officer (DRO) and the Employment Rehabilitation Service (ERS). However, changes within the Employment Service (ES) have seen the amalgamation of these services under a new system, PACT (Placement, Assessment and Counselling Team). One of the problems with PACTs is that they have to function with very little change to the system. The various packages and schemes on offer from PACT are much the same. Consequently it is necessary to review the schemes on offer before determining referral of a disabled employee for assessment. It may well be that an employer would choose to use an alternative assessment service specifically linked to the type of work he has to offer.

On 6th June 1994 a new programme for disabled people came into effect. Called Access to Work, its aim is to assist people who need help to overcome barriers to work resulting from disabilities. The new programme replaces and adds to the help previously available under Special Aids to Employment. People receiving help under the Personal Reader Service or Fares to Work were able to choose to remain on that scheme until 31st March 1995 or to transfer to Access to Work at any time from 6th June 1994. After 31st March 1995 those who remain on the original scheme automatically transfer to Access to Work. This means that assistance is no longer limited to prescribed specific forms, but that, within available resources, it provides flexibility to meet needs.

Access to Work is open to unemployed, employed or self-employed individuals registerable as disabled and is administered by PACTs. The programme offers funding up to £21 000 over five years (after five years the entitlement will begin again). Employers who wish to recruit someone with a disability, or to retain an already disabled or newly disabled employee, and who need help to do so, can bid for funding. They will not need to pay towards the cost unless the help under Access to Work brings additional benefits, e.g. the purchase of equipment that will also be used by non-disabled employees.

The Sheltered Placement Schemes (SPS), which evolved from sheltered workshops, are designed to help support disabled people within an integrated working environment. This is achieved via grant funding on an annual basis, which has an upper limit of £4000. Organizing such a scheme may involve setting up a contract with an outside body.

Where then is the main contribution of the occupational health professional in relation to retention and rehabilitation of the disabled employee?

Employment policies may need to be reviewed and revised, as appropriate, to enable rehabilitation of the employee with either a degenerating existing disability, a new disability, or indeed of a person suffering problems because of a change in the work process. Though many employers have a commitment to employing people with disabilities, very few it seems have the same commitment to retaining or even rehabilitating existing employees who develop long-term disabilities. This may be associated with statute, as with the Fire Service, where stringent standards for health are set down for fire-fighters. It is self-evident that fire-fighters should be fit in the interest of their own and others' safety, however, there are other jobs done in the Fire Service and there is the potential to retain some of these extremely skilled people. In other cases the problem is often associated with lack of proper advice and support for the employer. Most of all the employer needs to know 'how much of what' they can expect from the individual and how they might make adjustments to either the job or the workplace to get the best out of the disabled worker. The manager, the team and the disabled worker need to know what is planned, and what effect it will have on them individually and as a group. Success in rehabilitation is based on knowledge and confidence.

The occupational health professional can, and should, be an important player in the process of rehabilitation. Their knowledge of the workplace, production processes, health challenges and demands on individual employees or teams make them eminently suitable members of any group discussing rehabilitation of an employee. Their extended knowledge enables them to act as professional contact between the employee's own medical advisers and the employer. They are also able to advise on the use of external consultants should it be necessary, and are well placed to guide employers in the interpretation of the reports received from those consultants. In addition, they are best able, because of their duty to act as client advocate, to ensure a full understanding of client and employer needs as an outcome of rehabilitation.

The *Disability Rights Handbook* (Education and Research Association, 1993), which is published annually, is intended to act as an all-purpose rights guide for people with disabilities and their families. The *National Welfare Benefits Handbook* (Lakhani and Read, 1987/8) also published annually, is based on the experience of the workers and the Citizens' Rights Officer. Both are important publications for the occupational health professionals in that they offer a further support in the provision of informed advice for employees at a very difficult time in their lives.

WORK RELATED DISEASE AND REHABILITATION

Top of the scale of self-reported work related diseases are musculo-skeletal disorders. Back pain leads the list with almost half a million cases reported in 1990; when added together with all other cases (excluding RSI), the grand total was 891 000. However, the HSE annual report for 1990–91 estimated that only 61% of these cases were in fact 'caused' by work. The Loss Prevention Council also estimated a lower prevalence than reported, at some 535 000 cases. Second in estimated prevalence at 105 000 cases was stress/depression with 190 000 cases reported and 58% believed to be caused by work (Ballard, 1994b).

The problems associated with the high incidence in both these disease categories are related to the fact that they are more likely to cause frequent short-term absence rather than long-term absences in their early stages. Three to five days off work will often produce a sufficient reduction in symptoms for the worker to return to work only to be off again fairly soon. This not only exacerbates the causative factor, making each recurrence worse, but also makes achieving a resolution of the problem far more difficult. Not all of these diseases will be work related at their onset, but unless properly managed they will soon be categorized as 'made worse by work'.

In these cases early referral, early intervention and rehabilitation are the components for reduction in workplace health challenges. Worksite modification, job redesign or adaptation, aids and adaptations will all need to be considered if we are to reduce the effects of work on those suffering from these diseases. The involvement of physiotherapists and ergonomists in rehabilitation programmes for those with musculo-skeletal disorders will achieve more rapid resolution of the problem, though there is no guarantee of a cure. Those suffering from stress frequently need the support of an external consultant/counsellor but it must always be remembered that there is little value in 'treating only the casualty'. It is essential that the occupational health professional fully investigates the cause and the exacerbation factor, and applies his or her expertise to the reduction of risk of recurrence.

Rehabilitation of these employees is not easy. Managers and colleagues are never as supportive as when someone has been away long term and any change, no matter how essential, is always a challenge. The same care and attention should be given to the preparation and management of these cases as to the programme for the long-term sick returner.

Proper application of the Manual Handling Operations Regulations 1992 will help to reduce the future incidence of musculo-skeletal disorders.

The provision of a mental health policy will help in the management of those suffering from stress related disorders. A suggested format follows.

MENTAL HEALTH POLICY

1. Statement on mental health policy

1.1 ' .... ', recognizes that the workplace can be a stimulating and supportive environment and have a positive effect on mental health.

1.2 ' .... ' also recognizes that adverse situations can have a negative effect.

1.3 As a good employer, ' .... ' recognizes the need to promote Mental Health in a positive and pro-active manner.

1.4 The Mental Health Policy is seen as an enabling policy.

1.5 It is intended that this Policy will provide the framework for developing future positive policies which acknowledge organizational stress and other related disorders, and will be within the industrial relations framework.

2. Statement on mental health

2.1 Mental Health is a component of personal health and not a separate entity. If this is widely understood, apprehension about mental ill health will diminish.

2.2 Mental health problems do not necessarily prevent people from working.

2.3 Mental ill health creates a problem for the employer when it interferes with the effectiveness and working of the organization.

3. Aims

3.1 To promote mental health at work and help to prevent mental ill health.

3.2 To aid recognition of potential mental health problems.

3.3 To provide a basis for education and training.

3.4 To outline the processes of intervention and facilitate rehabilitation and resettlement at work after sickness absence, including as necessary, job design/redesign.

4. Objectives of the policy

4.1 To reduce the fear and apprehension about mental ill health and promote mental well-being.

4.2 To provide an information service for all employees.

4.3 To be applicable and useful to all individuals irrespective of their level of seniority.

4.4 To be acceptable to employees, management, unions and occupational health professionals.

4.5 To acknowledge that where the need to include external advice is necessary, that advice will be used.

4.6 To be capable of being adapted and applied into all departments of ' . . . . ', whatever the nature of the work and the resources available.

5. Resources planning

5.1 Training for Training Officers, Senior Managers, Managers, Supervisors, Personnel Officers and Union Stewards and Representatives.

5.2 Joint Management and Union Training in each sector is recommended to ensure both consistency and full use of functional resources.

5.3 Guidance notes will be developed to address the specific issues as and when these are identified.

ALCOHOL AND DRUG MISUSE

The larger the workplace the more likely it is to have some alcohol or 'sensible drinking' policy. Many such policies will incorporate drug and/or other substance misuse. There has been much research into the effect of substance misuse on the worker and the workplace; in a recent report alcohol misuse was estimated to cost industry some £2 billion a year (Maynard, 1992).

When developing systems to deal with the problems associated with excessive alcohol consumption it is essential to ensure that those systems can meet the needs of all employees at all levels of the company. A 1991 survey found that professional male workers (social class I) are over three times more likely to drink during working hours than unskilled male manual workers (social class V). There was a higher incidence of the effect of drink on work performance in young men whilst 4% of men and 2% of women admitted that they had been absent from work, with a hangover, at least once in the previous year (OPCS, 1991).

Specific training for managers and worker representatives probably plays the most important part in the management of substance misuse in the workplace. Early identification and early referral are the most effective method of achieving a resolution to what is undoubtedly a high risk behaviour in both health and safety terms. There will be 'failures' in the management of alcohol and other substance misuse cases but these appear to be getting fewer and fewer as occupational health professionals, working with other experts, influence change not only in the individual but in other workers and managers, other health care workers and in society generally.

The following is an example of a workplace policy for alcohol and drug misuse reduction:

ALCOHOL AND DRUG MISUSE POLICY

1. Statement on alcohol and drug misuse

1.1 As an employer, '. . . . . ' recognizes and accepts that nationally there is indisputable evidence to prove a growing alcohol and drug misuse (abuse) problem. Equally, as a good employer it sees itself as tackling this problem in a positive and preventive manner.

1.2 To fulfil the above, ' . . . . ' is to introduce an Alcohol and Drug Misue Policy. The information will be disseminated by means of education and training seminars, and the distribution of leaflets and the displaying of posters throughout the workplace.

2. Aim

The aim of the Alcohol and Drug Misuse Policy is to provide a framework in which to assist the employee to seek help advice and support, where applicable.

3. Objectives

3.1 To reduce alcohol and drug misuse through education and advice.

3.2 To ensure that management, personnel staff and trade union representatives are trained to recognize alcohol and drug-related problems early.

3.3 To ensure that referrals are made at the earliest possible time.

3.4 To ensure that all avenues where help can be found are known to employees.

3.5 To ensure absolute confidentiality.

3.6 To develop a training package that will be applicable to all areas of employment.

4. Statement of policy

4.1 This policy has been agreed jointly by the '. . . . . ' and those trade unions recognized by ' . . . . '.

4.2 Alcohol and drug misuse is recognized as a health and social problem and not normally a disciplinary matter, therefore people who misuse either require help and support.

4.3 Alcohol and drugs are a problem when a person takes them continually or repeatedly and the effects interfere with that person's health and/or job performance, or have an adverse reaction on others including family and colleagues at work.

4.4 It is '. . . . . ' intention to create an environment whereby employees who suspect or know that they have an alcohol or drugs problem are encouraged to seek help voluntarily.

4.5 The confidential nature of any records of employees with an alcohol or drugs problem (or other health problem) with be strictly preserved.

4.6 The policy is applicable to all employees irrespective of the position they hold and does not discriminate at any level.

5. Management of policy

5.1 Employees who come to notice, through observation or by normal procedures following poor work performance, as possibly having an alcohol or drug problem will be given the opportunity immediately to seek help. As few members of management or union representatives have the specific skills to provide this help, referrals should be via the departmental Occupational Health Nurse.

5.2 In all instances within items 4.4 and 5.1 the encouragement to seek and accept help is on the clear understanding that:
> The employee will be granted the necessary leave to seek help and support and such leave will be treated as sick leave. Every effort will be made to ensure that the employee after this period is able to return to the same job unless resumption of the same job would risk undermining a return to a satisfactory level of job performance.

5.3 Employees who, having come to notice as possibly having an alcohol or drug-related problem, either:
(a) decline to accept referral for help and support; or
(b) discontinue the course before its satisfactory completion; or
(c) continue to perform unsatisfactorily after treatment
will be monitored and reminded and, if appropriate, further opportunity will provided to accept and cooperate with help and support before any action under the usual recognized procedures.

5.4 This policy is not concerned with social drinking; the concern is limited to those instances of problem drinking which affect the work performance of the employee. The policy does not apply to employees who, because of excessive indulgence in alcohol or drugs on random occasions, behave in a manner contrary to the standards of safety and conduct required by ' . . . . ' – such instances will be dealt with in accordance with the normal and recognized disciplinary procedures.

EMPLOYEE ASSISTANCE PROGRAMMES

Where a return to his or her previous job is not possible, the worker will need advice regarding available options, counselling on managing the change, possibly identification of retraining needs and even, in extreme circumstances, 'out placement' support if he or she is to be retired on health grounds. No matter what the reason for the move, 'out placement' is in effect what is happening to the worker.

Employee Assistance Programmes (EAPs) are designed to provide confidential help, on a voluntary basis, to employees and immediate members of their family in order to deal with personal problems, some of which may be affecting their work performance. EAPs have been found to be cost effective in helping to reduce the costs of stress-related sickness absence. They are operated under the same ethical constraints with regard to confidentiality as apply to an occupational health unit.

In the main they provide a range of services which include advice related to alcohol and drugs; legal and financial concerns; work issues;

emotional concerns; family; marital and other relationships; smoking and eating disorders; care of the elderly, etc. They are able to take on wider roles and these may well extend into assessment, job application, retirement advice, etc. It is important that the providers of these services have a wide knowledge, not only of the processes of the company but of other employment opportunities in the neighbourhood.

Where referral to an EAP or similar service is being made it is essential that full details of any limitations caused by the individual's health status are clearly defined. Every effort should be made to ensure this report is written in 'lay' terms and that medical terminology is avoided.

Support for workers moving to other areas of employment or leaving employment completely is not wasted time. It helps to build a good relationship with both managers and other workers if the occupational health professional demonstrates an interest in the well-being of the workforce.

MULTIDIMENSIONAL HEALTH QUESTIONNAIRES

Many of the methods used to measure the health of employees do exactly that. They don't extend to asking clients how they feel. The use of multidimensional health measurement questionnaires has the potential to provide what is often the missing link in initial assessment and review of returners.

In the preface to a recent work, Ware writes: 'We are in an era during which health outcomes will increasingly be evaluated from the patient point of view. The benefits of specific treatments and of the health care delivery system in general will be judged in terms of the extent to which changes in the patient's functioning or well-being meet his or her needs and expectations' (Ware *et al.*, 1993).

Research conducted in the UK has shown that not all the health measurement questionnaires that have been produced are necessarily suitable for use in the UK let alone in an occupational health setting. For ease of use the occupational health professional will be looking for a short, simple to use, easily understood format that does not require complicated scoring mechanisms to interpret results. He or she will also wish to use data to demonstrate the effectiveness of interventions, and possibly, for research material. There must also be the ability to link occupational health and general practice outcomes with an acceptable degree of reliability. The process must be capable of validation. In addition because in the main occupational health professionals deal with healthy individuals, the health measurement questionnaire must be based on values derived from the general population and thus capable of demonstrating the norm for the workplace population. Finally, the questionnaire used (i.e. changes in health status) needs to be sensitive for lower levels of ill health if it is to be of value in the workplace.

Several health measurement questionnaires have been reviewed (Jenkinson, Wright and Coulter, 1993) including the Nottingham Health Profile (NHP), the Functional Limitations Profile (FLP), the Dartmouth Primary Care Co-operative Information Project (Co-op Project) and the Short Form-36 (SF-36).

The Co-op system, which is made up of nine illustrated charts, measures physical, social and role functioning, emotional status, social support, pain, quality of life, overall health and health change and is one of the easiest of these questionnaires to apply and score. The charts can be self completed in about five minutes and the results recorded immediately in the client's notes. They have been found to improve clinician/patient communication. However, the charts were not developed with the intention of using them in samples and populations, although they are reported to have been successfully used in this manner.

The SF-36 is the most well-known instrument to have come out of the USA's Medical Outcomes Study (MOS). It is short, and covers a wide range of areas that may be adversely affected by illness. It is sensitive to lower levels of disability and ill health (Brazier, Jones and Kind, 1992), though it does demonstrate a lower response rate among those over 65 years of age. The SF-36 measures physical functioning, social functioning, role limitations (physical), role limitations (emotional), mental health, energy/vitality, pain and general health perceptions. It can be self completed, used over a telephone or face to face by the clinician, and takes five minutes to complete. The wording of the American format has been slightly modified (i.e. Anglicized) for use in the UK, and is otherwise proving a most useful and acceptable instrument.

A further questionnaire, the Euroqol Instrument (EQ), was developed by a multidisciplinary group of researchers from five European centres (Brazier, Jones and Kind, 1993). Whilst the EQ measures much the same criteria as the SF-36, research to date has demonstrated that it is not capable of demonstrating less severe morbidity and is therefore, like the NHP and FLP, not likely to be the best instrument for use in occupational health settings.

At the time of writing the SF-36 appears to be the most acceptable health measurement questionnaire for use in occupational health practice. For its successful application, however, the occupational health practitioner will need to ensure its use in conjunction with demographic and work related information, thereby affording a broad range of data on which to base norms.

SCREENING FOR JOB PLACEMENT

In the past, pre-employment medical examinations have often been required by companies and carried out by doctors or other health professions without detailed enquiry into rationale (Smith, McGreggor and Rawll, 1992). This paper demonstrated the need for a rational approach to preplacement screening, setting standards of health and fitness for given work tasks. Once such criteria are developed and accepted by both management and workforce it is essential that the standard is applied to all job placements. This means that returners, redeployees and those being transferred or promoted into new posts should be health screened if the work task falls into such a category.

No single method of health screening will meet all the needs of an employer. The Management of Health and Safety at Work Regulations 1992 which came into force on 1st January 1993 introduced some new criteria for screening, and there is no doubt that as managers become more adept at conducting risk assessments, there will be an increased demand for the development or modification of health screening procedures.

For the returner, health screening will probably be seen as yet another challenge. It is beholden on the occupational health practitioner to ensure that the returner understands that this is a formal procedure related to health and safety requirements, applicable to any member of staff and not specifically designed for the purpose of health assessment for rehabilitation.

The use of the multidimensional health questionnaire, in conjunction with routine health screening procedures and linked to any other formal assessment, will afford a good understanding of the potential of the returner to carry out those tasks for which he or she is being rehabilitated.

NEGOTIATING REHABILITATION FOR WORK

It should be recognized that rehabilitation for work is not a simple process. Co-workers will have been affected by the absence of the returner; in some cases they will have had to take on extra work, work longer hours or modify the work process. In other situations relief staff will have been employed. In all cases there will have been changes. All of these elements need to be considered, especially if the absence has been in excess of six months. The work performance of the returner may have been poor prior to the period of absence and assurances may be needed that once rehabilitation has been achieved the equivalent work performance will be required from the returner as for all other similarly graded workers.

In some cases the concerns of the co-workers are associated with the diagnosed condition for absence. This is especially so when there has been a severe infection, when there is the risk of fits or collapse and when there is a history of mental ill health. Fear of infection with hepatitis or HIV is rarely found but certainly exists. Colleagues may be anxious or frightened at the thought of working alongside or being responsible for a person with a history of mental illness and/or fits. Here the occupational health nurse plays an important role by facilitating 'diagnosis' (Adolfsson, 1984) of the workgroup needs and creating a psychosocial environment of support and knowledge. The purpose of this work should be to prepare all the workers for potential challenges associated with the additional stressors the programme of rehabilitation may introduce, to inform the returner of the anxieties of colleagues and to advise on how best to address those anxieties, and to give the occupational health nurse the opportunity to come into close contact with the people who will eventually form the returner's 'support group'.

Initially the occupational health nurse will need to seek the written, informed consent of the returner to discuss his or her particular case with his or her colleagues. The returner may choose to lead the initial 'information giving' meeting, with the occupational health nurse acting as advocate and facilitator. However, in practice, this event usually takes place much later in the process. In this circumstance the occupational health nurse will lead the initial information-giving session when, having been given consent, he or she will describe the condition and explain its effect prior to treatment, its effect following or with treatment and the expected prognosis. Where consent for full disclosure has not been obtained a more general information session will have to be sufficient. It is essential that colleagues understand the limitations placed on the returner and the type of support that will be needed from them. When the absence has been longer than six weeks there is value in asking them to list any workplace and personal changes that the returner may not be aware of, i.e. new work programme, changes in mileage allowances, someone's become engaged, a new manager, someone's left, etc. They need to understand as much as the returner that things have 'moved on' since he or she went off sick.

A few days after the initial information session a further meeting should be arranged for considered questions to be asked and for clarification of any specific factors for all participants in the process. Following this the occupational health nurse and manager will negotiate the phased return to work programme with the returner and arrange a start date. At this meeting the first 'check up' date should be set, usually for about two weeks into the programme. This 'check up' can be conducted by the manager who can call on the occupational health nurse if necessary.

The second 'check up' should involve the occupational health nurse in a review of the returner's health status and if necessary in the setting up of a final group session to analyse the process and to afford feedback. This is frequently one of the most supportive elements of the process and presents a forum for the returner and occupational health nurse to thank colleagues for their support.

PHASED RETURN TO WORK

A process for achieving early return to work is an important element of any rehabilitation programme. If properly designed such a process can lead to better management of the returnee, giving him or her the support needed and offering permanency to that return. Colleagues are much more supportive of individuals when they are involved in a structured return to work.

The following programme is currently being assessed as part of an absence reduction programme.

PHASED RETURN TO WORK

1. Introduction

1.1 In order to more successfully rehabilitate employees back into the workplace following long-term ill health a 'phased return to work scheme' has been introduced.

1.2 The scheme is funded by individual departments.

2. Aims

2.1 The aims are not only to achieve an earlier return to work but also to afford permanency to that return.

2.2 Rehabilitation is to be the most important factor.

2.3 A flexible approach controlled by the client/patient, his or her general practitioner/consultant and the occupational health nurse.

2.4 To enable/support job redesign/adaptation and/or redeployment/ training, or retraining the worker to cope with the pressure of a full return to work.

2.5 To provide additional services to those provided by the Department of Employment and, where necessary, to link those services.

3. Methodology

3.1 Initial contact is made by the occupational health nurse (OHN) following referral from any source.

3.2 The OHN negotiates with the client and his/her general practitioner and/or consultant the timing and method of achieving a 'phased return'.

3.3 The OHN then recommends the method of return to the manager and personnel section.

3.4 Until such time as the general practitioner and OHN agree that the hours worked are in excess of hours away from work the client will be supervised jointly by the general practitioner and OHN.

3.5 The OHN and manager will supervise the remainder of the programme.

3.6 There will be an OHN review prior to full working and following a period of full working.

4. Suggested programme

4.1

	Monday	Tuesday	Wednesday	Thursday	Friday
Week 1	off	pm only	off	pm only	off
Week 2	am only	off	pm only	off	am only
Week 3	am only	pm only	am only	pm only	am only
Week 4	1/2 day	full day	1/2 day	full day	1/2 day
Week 5	full day	1/2 day	full day	1/2 day	full day
Week 6	Full Time Working Week				
Week 7	Return To Normal Work Pattern				

4.2 In some cases there may be a need to adopt more flexibility in the time element allocated at the start of the programme (i.e. first three weeks).

4.3 In many cases a full return to work will be achieved in less time.

CONCLUSION

Rehabilitation for work needs to start as soon as possible after notification of an accident or of ill health. Procedures need to be developed in conjunction with management and worker representatives. Consultation should take place with PACTs, general practitioners and other external consultants prior to setting up the procedures and developing policy.

The ability of the occupational health professional to assist with rehabilitation and redeployment provides not only a cost effective way to reduce absence but an all encompassing demonstration of the employer's contribution to the well-being of the workforce.

CASE STUDY 1

Mary had previously diagnosed as a schizophrenic 14 years but, apart from occasional absences from work for various ill health problems, had maintained regular attendance and performed all her duties reasonably well. Her work as a general office clerk was mundane and not particularly challenging, even for Mary, though she'd never sought any promotion or job change. None of her work colleagues knew of her diagnosis; she wasn't registered disabled for work.

Suddenly Mary began to behave strangely at work: she started accusing staff of saying things about her, she hid documents, misfiled others, wasn't as careful with her appearance and was often late for work. When challenged by her line manager she could be quite aggressive. She had been formally advised that her behaviour, time-keeping and appearance were not acceptable. She was now considered almost unemployable and would therefore be dismissed if she failed to improve on all counts. Her trade union representative asked for an occupational health opinion.

Following that referral contact was made with Mary's general practitioner who agreed to see her and discuss re-referral to her erstwhile consultant. Mary was signed off work long-term sick and was visited at home by her occupational health nurse. It was agreed that the nurse would attend the outpatient appointment with Mary and that they would discuss the problems at work with her consultant. It was also agreed that Mary would register 'Disabled for Work' which would offer some protection to her continued employment on a reasonable salary.

Mary's health problems had come to light when her sister, with whom she had lived for most of her adult life, moved away and left Mary in their shared home with only occasional visits from family and friends. Previously Mary had taken her medication regularly because it was less fuss than having an argument with her sister. She'd always believed it wasn't necessary, and since she'd been alone she'd proved she didn't need it. Mary couldn't recognize the change in herself; she was very anxious but felt that things would be better when people stopped blaming her for everything. She was not suffering from any ill health and should be allowed to return to work. The neighbours were ganging up on her and she didn't care. She knew her parents were frightened of her and she didn't want her sister near her. Mary was admitted to hospital under the Mental Health Act 1983.

Rehabilitation for Mary was a protracted business. It involved regular visits to hospital by the occupational health nurse and, following some resolution of her symptoms, gradual resocialization with some of her work colleagues. Following her discharge from hospital, and with her consent, Mary's community psychiatric nurse (CPN) and the occupational health nurse set up and ran an awareness seminar for Mary's work colleagues. This was well accepted and Mary's 'phased return to work' was negotiated with her manager, consultant and CPN, who spoke with her general practitioner about the planned programme. Prior to the start of the phased return to work programme the occupational health nurse met once again with the workplace team and asked them to consider what changes had taken place during Mary's absence and to list any such changes. They were surprised at how much change there had been in the four months Mary had been away.

Mary's return was very gradual: only two half days a week for two weeks and it was five weeks before she achieved attendance for some part of every day for a full working week. The effort put in by the staff to normalize work for Mary was marvellous. They say it was easy because they knew what to do, what had happened to Mary and what her illness could do to her. However, once Mary was again assimilated into the workplace and into society generally they placed a requirement on Mary. With the support of the occupational health nurse Mary was able to meet that requirement. She spoke to her colleagues about schizophrenia, about her illness and the treatment she was currently taking. She asked them to tell her if she seemed unwell and if she wasn't doing her work properly.

That was six years ago. Since then Mary has been a productive team member. There have been occasional slippages but, as Mary would tell you herself, she hasn't 'gone off the boil'. There is no formal review procedure arranged with the occupational health nurse, though Mary does confirm her biannual re-registration as 'Disabled for Work'.

CASE STUDY 2

Asif had threatened a number of tenants with a machete in the block of flats where he was a caretaker. This was not an isolated incident over the past 12 months and it prompted disciplinary action. No doubt it would have resulted in his eventual dismissal had not the trade union representative asked for an independent assessment of Asif's behaviour, a course of action which was backed by the occupational health nurse.

The line manager was given responsibility for coordination and an initial meeting involving Asif, trade union disability officer and occupational health nurse decided to ask for the advice of a specialist consultant.

The result of the assessment which included medical and social background as well as occupational psychology testing was of immense interest. It showed Asif to be in the top 2% of the population on intelligence quotients covering literacy and mathematical tests. It revealed that Asif had had schizophrenia for many years, managed successfully by medication, until it altered 12 months ago. Finally it showed a man in a degree of social isolation both within his own culture and that of his adopted one. His perceived lack of status simply exacerbated the problem.

In discussion with his doctor, the consultant and of course Asif, the medication was reassessed resulting in a return to reasonable behaviour. Redeployment was negotiated within the Housing Department into a post which offered possibilities of advancement, i.e. benefits assistance, a move which pleased Asif.

The cost to the Department added up to time, thought and a few hundred pounds for outside help. In return they gained a committed and enthusiastic employee.

(Whitfield, 1993a)

CASE STUDY 3

Helen worked at a main reception point not because this was what she was good at, though she was, but because this was the only post she felt she could manage because of her failing sight. Management did not view it as an issue until financial stringencies indicated the possibility of redundancies. Both Helen and her line manager were confronted with changes which they did not really want to acknowledge since Helen could 'pass' as normal since she did not look disabled (*sic*). This self-imposed barrier had prevented them from exploring options in the past which would have aided Helen's career development and increased her value as an employee.

With the help of the PACT team Helen, as a starting point, was provided with some LUNA software to install on the computer used by Helen's team. This system expanded the text on the screen and allowed Helen to renew word processing skills in which she already had some training. It also allowed her to disseminate information that much more efficiently.

This simple solution helped Helen to be viewed as a more valued team member and integrated her in a more real sense than previously.

(Whitfield, 1993b)

CASE STUDY 4

Susan is in her 20s and had worked as a nursery nurse in the the UK and in Pakistan. She was working in a social work department in the latter when she became ill in March 1987.

'During March of that year I caught what appeared at first to be a cold. Within a couple of days I thought it must be flu and had a few days off work. Daily I became worse and each trip to the local hospital produced a different diagnosis and a new explanation as to why I was not recovering.

'I slept for the best part of the first two months. When I was up again I brought a typewriter home from the office along with some of the more routine work. When I was feeling a little stronger I desperately wanted to get back to work. The offices were on a compound with living accommodation so I would drive into the city with my flatmate, work for maybe an hour or so until coffee break and then go to bed until lunch. I'd work a bit more and then go back to bed for another sleep. The number of days I worked varied from one week to the next and this pattern continued for the first year or so. Eighteen months after the start of my illness, which was eventually diagnosed as ME (myalgic encephalomyelitis), I returned to the UK. I took three months off and was beginning to feel much better and took a part-time job with a local solicitor. Almost two years after the initial infection

I felt ready to go back to work full time. I took another job commuting into London. After two months this was clearly too much and I had to take time off and then go back to working part time. I found a local job with the ME Association which is very flexible. I feel that my employment options have been restricted and are still very limited. I cannot envisage going back into the profession I was trained for in the immediate future. I am very aware that had I not been given the opportunity to return to work on such a flexible basis I could still be unemployed.'

(Hawkes and Paschkes Bell, 1993)

CASE STUDY 5

David worked as manager of a branch of a major financial institution.

'My health had been deteriorating for a year; the GP diagnosed a sinus problem and "stress". I then collapsed and was admitted to hospital where a brain tumour was diagnosed. I underwent surgery and radiotherapy and was able to return to work 11 months later. My main residual problem was short-term memory loss, due to the tumour haemorrhaging.

'My employers told me that because of this and my long absence from work I could not return to my former management level job. Although the organization was initially helpful, no effort was made to establish with my medical specialists the best working environment for me and for months I was pushed around a number of branches doing odd tasks with no regular routine, the worst possible situation for me. When the recession forced a "headcount reduction" programme I received a redundancy notice.

'My trade union stepped in to help. The union brought my case to the attention of specialist staff in the institution's personnel department who were extremely helpful and supportive. Soon afterwards I was offered a job at one of their security processing centres and the threat of redundancy was lifted. A full assessment of my memory disability was made by an independent specialist charity and the Disablement Advisory Service* supplied me with an electronic organizer to supplement my short-term memory.

'I feel my case would have been helped if I had been assessed earlier and if my employer had received advice on the optimum working environment for me; this would have spared me con-

> siderable anxiety and enabled me to have achieved a full work contribution much sooner.'
> *Phased out in 1992 in favour of PACTs
>
> *(Hawkes and Paschkes Bell, 1993)*

REFERENCES

Adolfsson, A. (1984) *Efficiency, Working Environment, Health*, Bygghalsan, Stockholm, Sweden.

Audit Commission (1990) *Managing Sickness Absence in London*, HMSO, London.

Ballard, J. (1994a) Actions on health – HSE policy statement. *Occupational Health Review*, **48**, 24–7.

Ballard, J. (1994b) ILL health data – Just where to begin? *Occupational Health Review*, **48**, 17–18.

Brazier, J.E., Harper, R., Jones, N.M.B. *et al.* (1992) Validating the SF-36 health survey questionnaire: new outcome measure for primary care. *British Medical Journal*, **305**, 160–4.

Brazier, J., Jones, N. and Kind, P. (1993) Testing the validity of Euroqol and comparing it with the SF-36 health survey questionnaire. *Quality of Life Research*, (2) 169–80.

Education and Research Association (1993) *Disability Rights Handbook*, The Disability Alliance, London, UK.

Hawkes, J. and Paschkes Bell, G. (1993) *Disability Leave – A Guide for Employers*, Royal National Institute for the Blind, London, UK.

Health and Safety Commission (1992) *Management of Health and Safety at Work: Approved Code of Practice*, HSE Books, Sudbury, UK.

Jenkinson, C., Wright L. and Coulter, A. (1993) *Quality of Life Measurement in Health Care*, Health Service Research Unit, Oxford, UK.

Lakhani, B. and Read, J. (1987/88) *National Welfare Benefits Handbook*, Child Poverty Action Group, London, UK.

Maynard, M. (1992) *Social Costs of Alcohol*, Centre for Health Economics, York.

Nygren, A., *et al.* (1993) Rehabilitation of patients with neck and shoulder pain – impact on sickness absence from work. Paper presented at 24th Congress of the International Commission on Occupational Health, Nice, France (unpublished).

OPCS (1991) *Drinking in England and Wales in the late 1980s*, Office of Population Censuses and Surveys, London, UK.

Paschkes Bell, G.P. and Wavell, Z. (1990) *Feasibility Study into Future Provision of RNIB Rehabilitation Services in England, Wales and Northern Ireland 1989/90*, Royal National Institute for the Blind, London, UK.

Smith, K., McGreggor, A.R. and Rawll, C. (1992) Screening for Job Placement: an in-house placement screening programme. *Occupational Medicine*, **42**, 64–8.

Ware, J.E., Snow, K.K., Kosinski, M. and Gandek, B. (1993) *SF-36 Health Survey – Manual and Interpretation Guide*, New England Medical Centre, Boston, USA.

Whitfield, D. (1993a) *Retaining Disabled Employees – A Manager's Guide*, Metropolitan Authorities Recruitment Agency, London, UK.

Whitfield, D. (1993b) *Retaining Disabled Employees – Creating a Policy and Supporting a Strategy*, Metropolitan Authorities Recruitment Agency, London, UK.

FURTHER READING

Aitken, R.C.B. and Cornes, P. (1990) To work or not to work: that is the question. *British Journal of Industrial Medicine*, **47**, 436–41.

Audit Commission (1993) *Get Well Soon*, HMSO, London, UK.

Ballard, J. (1993) Workers' Compensation: a case study of America's largest insurer. *Occupational Health Review*, **43**, 17–21.

Employment Service (1994) *Access to Work*, Employment Department, London, UK.

Employment Service (1994) *Disabled People and Work*, Employment Department, London, UK.

Hamblin, P.M. (1993) *Help to Hand*, Nurse Practitioner Services Ltd, London.

Hunter, J. (1989) Commentary on vocational rehabilitation in Great Britain. *Canadian Journal of Rehabilitation*, **2**(3), 131–6.

Jenkins, R. (1993) Mental health at work – why is it so under-researched? *Occupational Medicine*, **43**, 65–7.

Jenkinson, C. and Wright, L. (1993) The SF-36 Health Survey Questionnaire. *Auditorium*, **2**, 7–12.

Kennedy, M.S. (1986) Able to work? *Occupational Therapy*, 354–6.

Reid, W.M. and Smith, S.E. (1993) Elements of a comprehensive absenteeism control program. *American Association of Occupational Health Nurses Journal*, **41**(2), 90–5.

Thompson, D. and Pudney, M. (1990) *Mental Illness: The Fundamental Facts*, Mental Health Foundation, London, UK.

Waldron, H.A. (1989) *Occupational Health Practice*, Butterworths, London, UK.

Diseases of occupations

5

Kit Artus

A BRIEF HISTORY

The history of occupational disease is closely related to the perceptions, conscience and sophistication of the capitalist societies. For example, in ancient times the miners were primarily slaves, criminals or prisoners, so the labour force was easily replaced and the work was considered a punishment. Concern regarding the miners' disabilities or demise was therefore of little import.

Agricola (1494–1555) and Paracelsus (1493–1541) recorded the first observations on miners and their related diseases. As mining changed in the Middle Ages to deeper mines the incidence of respiratory diseases became more evident. Eventually miners organized themselves into societies and provided some social benefits such as sickness benefit and funeral expenses (Rosen, 1943).

In 1700 Ramazzini (1633–1714) published the first study of diseases related to trades, *De Morbis Artificum Diatriba*. He is recognized as the father of occupational medicine and was the first to advise physicians to seek information about the patient's occupation, a question still valid today. He identified two types of workplace hazards: the harmful character of materials handled, and certain violent and irregular motions and unnatural postures of the body, by reason of which the natural structure of the vital machine is so impaired that serious diseases gradually develops.

During the Industrial Revolution society and the countryside changed as the manufacture and production of goods was centralized in factories. Families moved to towns to obtain work and as a consequence the rural population declined. Overcrowding, poor housing, exposure to toxic chemicals at work, poor public health, pollution and social deprivation were commonplace. The demand for factory labour continued apace. The new machinery was capable of maiming as well as producing much sought after goods. The unguarded machines demanded nimble hands and feet working in cramped conditions in, around and under machinery. Employers paid low wages, housing and food had to be purchased, instead of grown, so all members of the family had to earn. Children were employed or sold to mill owners in their thousands. The poor conditions continued without control until 1802 when the 'Act for the preservation of the Health and Morals of Apprentices, and others employed in cotton and other mills and cotton and other factories' was introduced (Charley, 1954).

There were some worthy people working to increase the awareness of society of the plight of the common man and his family. In 1824 the Combination Acts of 1799 and 1800 were repealed. The importance of this change was immediately apparent from the number of unions which organized and exerted influence for the reduction of hours of work and an increase in wages. Later they turned their interest to health and safety, sustained to the present time (Schilling, 1981).

In 1831 Charles Thackray published *The Effects of the Principal Arts, Trades and Professions on Health.* It is apparent from the literature that the employment and exploitation of children was still a social issue. Eventually the concerned public became interested in the effects on children of working in appalling conditions. In 1833 a Factories Enquiry Commission was established which resulted in the first factory act in 1833. The Act was described as an 'Act to regulate the labour of children and young persons in mills and factories'.

The Factories Act 1833 required:

1. The appointment of four inspectors to cover the 3000 factories. The inspectors replaced the visitors appointed under the 1802 Factory Act and they could impose fines on the spot.
2. The minimum age of employment was nine years and no person under 18 to work more than 10 hours per day. No person under 21 to work at night.
3. Children from ages nine to 13 to attend school for 12 hours per week.
4. Industry was to establish day schools.
5. Children between nine and 13 years were not to be employed in a factory without a certificate of physical ability issued from a certifying surgeon.

The Factory Act of 1844 gave inspectors powers to appoint certifying surgeons. This was intended to prevent parents taking their children from one surgeon to another until they obtained a certificate of physical ability. Such was the need for employment for the whole family to survive that parents shifted from feeding their children gin to keep them small, so that they could move easily around the machinery, to giving them infusions of indigo to make them appear older.

The Registration of Births Act 1837 led to the certifying surgeons becoming redundant as the age of employees could be ascertained and the need for a certificate of physical ability was no longer a requirement for employment.

Another milestone of social improvement was the Public Health Act 1848. Awareness of the relevance of work, public health and education as means of essential social change and improvement was beginning to become apparent to Victorian society. A year after the crowning of Queen Victoria the Education Act of 1839 was placed on the statute books. The Factory Act of 1855 created new responsibilities for the certifying surgeons. They were to certify that young people were not incapacitated for work by disease or physical infirmity, and were responsible for investigating industrial accidents.

Towards the end of the nineteenth century, workers in certain dangerous trades were examined by the certifying surgeons due to the requirement to notify important industrial diseases. The duty to investigate notified cases of industrial disease was placed on the certifying surgeons who had the powers to suspend the sufferer from work. The results of this work eventually led to the appointment of the first Medical Inspector of Factories – T.M. Legge (1863–1932).

The voluntary appointment of doctors by employers followed the passing of the Workmen's Compensation Act 1897. The appointments were primarily a protective measure against claims for damages from the employers.

At times of war nations need their people to be fit for service in the fighting forces. In 1915 the Health of Munitions Workers' Committee was established which funded scientific research into the effects of munitions work on the health of employees. A recognition of required action led to the introduction of first aid, industrial medicine and nursing. This commitment to developing services for employees was not sustained after the war due to a downturn in the economy and resultant high unemployment. However, the principles and benefits of a healthy workforce were established.

The state continued to provide a statutory medical service through the Appointed Factory Doctors supervised by Medical Inspectors of Factories. The Appointed Factory Doctors had three main duties:

1. to examine young persons under the age of 18 for fitness to work and to re-examine them annually;
2. to periodically examine persons engaged in certain dangerous trades;
3. to investigate and report on notifiable diseases or injuries due to exposure to noxious substances.

This service continued until the introduction of the Employment Medical Advisory Service in 1972.

The Health and Safety at Work etc. Act 1974 changed the emphasis of health and safety legislation. This Act introduced consultation, rights of safety representatives, general concepts of health, safety and welfare, provision of information, instruction, training and supervision and a gradual shift away from the prescriptive control of the Factories Acts, the Offices, Shops and Railway Premises Acts and other Statutory Instruments.

The response of commerce and industry to the Health and Safety at Work etc. Act 1974 was often directed towards safety with too little reference to health beyond the personnel issues of pre-employment health surveillance, fitness to work and early retirement due to ill health. The European Union and the following health and safety regulations have focused awareness on the need to direct attention to the prevention of work related diseases and ill health. The requirement for workplace risk assessments can be seen to support the trend towards self-regulation.

SOURCES OF INFORMATION ON DISEASES OF OCCUPATION

There are numerous sources of information available to study the extent of occupational disease in the UK, e.g. Occupational mortality – the Registrar General's Decennial Supplement for Great Britain; the Department for Social Services Industrial Injuries Schemes (DSS II); the Health and Safety Commission Reports (HSC), etc. However, it is difficult for those involved in occupational health and safety practice to compare data as the sources are varied, the data is presented differently and recently there have been significant changes to recording periods. To further confuse the situation from October 1986 Injury and Disablement Benefit was changed to Disablement Benefit and compensation is now paid only for cases with a disability assessed at 14% or more.

There have been some additions to the prescribed diseases list – a list of diseases which, if diagnosed and if the sufferer is or has been employed in the specified occupations or activities, allow a claim can be submitted for Disablement Benefit through the Industrial Injuries Schemes (II) administered by the Department of Social Security (DSS). The additional diseases are:

- Occupational asthma – benefit first payable from 1982
- Lung cancer (asbestos) – benefit first payable from 1985
- Bilateral pleural thickening – benefit first payable from 1985
- Vibration white finger – benefit first payable from 1984/85.

These conditions are also reportable under The Reporting of Injuries,

Diseases and Dangerous Occurrences Regulations 1985 (Health and Safety Commission Annual Report, 1990/91).

The Reporting of Injuries, Diseases and Dangerous Occurrences Regulations 1985 (RIDDOR) is deficient as it does not require employers to report all current significant occupational diseases. Another dimension to reporting and hence investigation by the enforcement authorities is that conditions caused by cumulative strain are often not perceived as fitting the definition of accident in RIDDOR and as a consequence may not be reported. This employer rationale can be extended to conditions due to microtrauma such as work related upper limb disorder (WRULD) and back pain. The Health and Safety Commission recognize the difficulties that the changes and limited list of reportable diseases cause. However, the end result is under-reporting and, as a consequence, the risk of significant delays in eliminating the causes of disease and subsequent health benefits to employees and the population at large.

Recently two additional sources of data relating to occupational disease have been introduced – Surveillance of Work Related and Occupational Disease (SWORD) and EPIDERM (for 'epidermis') to monitor cases of dermatitis. The new schemes obtain information from specialists who identify and report cases which are probably occupational in origin. The number of cases reported from the two main sources varies widely: taking the most extreme of examples – the DSS II for Respiratory Diseases diagnosed 553 cases of occupational asthma, SWORD diagnosed 1047 cases. For dermatitis the DSS II figure is 411 cases and for EPIDERM the number is 2636 cases (1993 provisional) (Health and Safety Commission Annual Report, 1992/93). The annual figure of 2636 cases of dermatitis was calculated on reports from 50% of UK consultants in the first three months of the project.

Some comfort can be gained from the downward or static trend of the traditional occupational diseases. However, other conditions are showing an upward trend.

- Asbestosis and mesothelioma – cases and death benefit awards are still rising, reflecting the long latent period between exposure and diagnosis of disease. The estimated number of deaths due to asbestosis and related diseases is nearing 3000 annually. The number of new cases of asbestosis diagnosed by the Industrial Injuries Special Medical Boards in 1990–91 nearly doubled. Of concern is the number of new cases arising after the introduction of The Control of Asbestos at Work Regulations 1987 which set controls for asbestos levels based on the 4 hour and 10 minute Time Weighted Averages (TWAs).
  Of particular concern is the increasing number of cases of

mesothelioma in the younger age group. Over 1000 deaths were recorded for mesothelioma in 1992, a 15% rise on 1990.

- Pneumoconiosis – cases have remained steady at around 400 cases per year since 1984.
- Occupational asthma – numbers assessed under the DSS II for occupational asthma continue to grow. The SWORD scheme identified over 1000 cases in 1992 (1047 in 1993). This demonstrates that not all cases are being identified by the requirement to report under RIDDOR. Public concern and awareness continues to grow as the number of children suffering the illness appears to be increasing.
- Occupational deafness – claims appears to have declined to 972 cases in 1992 from 1128 cases in 1991.
- Vibration white finger – new cases peaked in 1991/92 to 5401 but have fallen back to 2369 cases in 1992/93.
- Musculo-skeletal problems – including the narrow range of accepted conditions such as tenosynovitis, upper limb cramp and sub-cutaneous cellulitis conditions are increasing. However, there is a large number of noncompensatable cases which are not monitored but are reported to the patient's general practitioner (Health and Safety Commission Annual Report, 1992/93).

It is salutary to note that there were reported to the HSE (all industries):

- 326 fatal injuries to employees and 84 fatal injuries to the self-employed in 1990/91;
- 249 fatal injuries to employees and 60 fatal injuries to the self-employed in 1992/93.

However, the data for deaths due to occupational disease in 1987 was 927 (Industrial Death Benefits all schemes). Death Benefit is not payable after 10th April 1988 and 1987 is the last full year of data from this source (source: DSS). Deaths due to occupational lung diseases reported in 1992 were 1491 (taken from 1991 death certificates).

Other new cases of occupational diseases diagnosed and assessed under the DSS II totalled 1904 cases and from RIDDOR 189 cases (Health and Safety Commission Annual Report, 1992/93).

The Employment Department's 1990 Labour Force Survey (LFS) (Health and Safety Commission Annual Report 1992/93 Statistical Supplement) identified that around 750 000 workers took time off work in 1989/90 because of what they believed were work related illnesses. A further 730 000 people believed that they had a work related illness but took no time off work. Some 820 000 retired or unemployed people reported that they were suffering from long-term work related illnesses.

The largest groups of illnesses reported were musculo-skeletal, hearing loss, stress/depression and lower respiratory disease. It is also reported that work related diseases account for about 7% of general practitioner (GP) consultations by people of working age. This was confirmed by a survey (Central Statistical Office, 1987) by the Employment Medical Advisors (EMAS) which found that 6% of GP consultations were for work related diseases.

It is apparent from this cursory study of some of the readily available data that the true incidence of occupational disease is still hidden and of a greater extent than death or disability caused by accidents. The pessimist may believe that some employers still bias their investment in safety to the detriment of the real problems of the 1990s – that of diseases of occupation.

The Health and Safety Commission Annual Report 1992/93 declares occupational health to be a priority. The intent is essentially to identify the main areas of occupational health needs to improve the employees' health related to occupations and to establish a means to identify ways of linking this work with the government initiatives declared in the document *The Health of The Nation* (Department of Health, 1991).

In the same report the Health and Safety Executive (HSE) found that:

1. half the workforce is in establishments using health professionals;
2. use of occupational hygienists has grown significantly since 1976;
3. most (65%) private sector employers take action to protect workers' health;
4. health hazards most commonly recognized were manual handling, chemicals, visual display units (VDUs), and work and dust/fumes.

THE HEALTH OF THE NATION

The government initiative *The Health of the Nation* (Department of Health, 1991) was welcomed by the majority of health professionals. The five key areas identified in the publication for directed concentration of effort cover coronary heart disease and stroke, cancers, mental illness, accidents, HIV/AIDS and sexual health, and cannot be considered unnecessary. However, when one considers that people spend one-third of their life at work it is a pity that a sixth key area of reduction – diseases of occupations – was omitted, particularly when you consider the financial and human costs of disease of occupation:

- in excess of 1.5 million people directly affected by diseases of occupation;
- 7% of GP consultations;
- 24% of causes of absence from work (including holidays);
- 13 million days off work per annum;
- costing up to £9 billion per annum = 10% of total company profits (exclusive of low performance and compensation).

The omission of occupational diseases is particularly disappointing as previous health promotion initiatives, such as the Look after your Heart campaign, were perceived by employers as being of benefit to the employers' objectives of reduction of absence from work attributed to ill health. Certainly health promotion is gaining importance in companies who have health professionals but the continuing separation of health at work from high profile national campaigns can be seen as a lost opportunity for the directed reduction of diseases of occupation through an informed workforce.

WHAT IS OCCUPATIONAL DISEASE?

Occupational disease can be defined as acute and chronic ill health caused by physical, ergonomic, chemical or biological agents as well as adverse effects on mental health. The diagnosis, identification of causes and the subsequent control of risk to reduce occupational disease are complex. There is recognition that the challenges to preventing occupationally induced diseases are subtle. The period between exposure and diagnosis of disease can be as long as 30 years. The increasing use of chemicals, their impact on the environment and exposure to combinations of chemicals have extended beyond the work environment to the population at large. The employer, employee, public exposure and perception of risk are a challenge for generations to come.

The well defined diseases of occupation resulting from exposure to specified substances such as asbestos, chemicals, silica, respiratory sensitizers, ionizing radiation, etc. are well understood, being the basis of regulatory health surveillance. However, most of the damage caused by work is similar to and interacts with the ill health caused by other life activities. The question often asked is 'How to identify the diseases and conditions caused by work and not by lifestyle or non-work activities?' The cause and effect argument is blurred as the health of the population is the sum total of work and social factors. Respiratory problems and disability due to musculo-skeletal problems are common in the population generally. Of equal significance is the lack of awareness by employees of the possibility that common symptoms are being caused by work activities or exposure to environmental contamination in the workplace. Examples of this may be vibration white finger, which some sufferers put down to poor circulation, and asthma, which appear to be increasing in the population at large. Is the cause of asthma environmental pollution at work, the general environment, better diagnosis or some other factor(s)? These questions are now being debated.

The current high level of unemployment, the lack of job security, the hectic lifestyle, the dual roles of working women, machine paced work, isolation, harassment and discrimination are escalating the debate about the responsibilities of employers in the area of psychosocial factors at work. Stress and stress-related diseases are recognized as contributing to the incidence of digestive problems, cardiovascular disease and mental ill health. Society generally is seeing dramatic changes at a time when organizations are also changing. In all areas of life there is increasing stress; the experience of change and the individual inability to manage change are adding to stress at home and at work.

The health professionals are slowly introducing the holistic approach to care. There is a growing recognition of the multi-faceted nature of ill health due to a general decline of the health of major sectors of society, an ageing population, unemployment and diseases of lifestyle and occupation. Employers are having to take a broader view of the risks to health created by employment and the problems of an ageing workforce. There is a recognition of the financial limits to health funding in response to, in particular, the ageing population and the sophistication of health technology; as a consequence the government is beginning to address the whole issue of health and health care.

DISEASES OF OCCUPATION AND TOXICOLOGY

Paracelsus (1493–1541) wrote, 'All substances are poisons: there are none which is not a poison. The right dose differentiates a poison and a remedy'. The modern day approach to toxicology is the quantitative study of the body's response to a substance.

A fundamental principle of toxicology is that all substances can kill if received by an inappropriate route and/or in sufficient quantities, e.g. drowning. The occupational health practitioner cannot be expected to be a toxicologist, however the Control of Substances Hazardous to Health Regulations 1988 (COSHH) (HSC, 1993) and the need to reduce the risks to health caused by exposure to substances, require an understanding of the basic principles of the hazards and risks presented by substances that employees are exposed to at the workplace. In other words, a sufficient knowledge of the principles of toxicology is needed to advise on the implementation of risk assessment programmes and the interpretation of these results to meet the requirements of COSHH and to protect the health of those exposed.

The number of chemicals in use in the UK is estimated to be between 40 000 and 100 000. Over 90% of these do not have a minimal toxicity test under the Notification of New Substances Regulations 1993 and there are no chronic toxicity tests for over 70% of these chemicals.

There were 156 236 deaths due to cancer in the UK in 1985 (Central Statistical Office, 1987). It is estimated that between 2% and 8% (excluding mesothelioma and bladder cancer) could be attributed to occupational exposure which could mean there were between 2600 and 10 400 cancer deaths due to occupational exposure (Doll and Peto, 1985). Other sources estimate that up to 30% of cancers are due to occupational exposure.

Substances may enter the body via several routes:

1. Inhalation is the most common and efficient route.
2. Skin absorption is more common than is appreciated particularly if the material is fat-soluble. The Health and Safety Executive (HSE) annual publication *Occupational Exposure Limits* notes the risk of skin absorption – 'Sk'.
3. Ingestion is unusual in the workplace but may follow from inhaled particles returned via the ciliary escalator or accidentally due to a breakdown in safe systems of work.
4. Accidental injection of a substance is a low risk but can occur as a result of a penetrating injury caused by a contaminated object, e.g. beryllium which can cause granuloma. This accidental injection is an inevitable risk in the health care sector due to frequent handing of sharps – instruments and needles – and subsequent accidental injection of pathogenic organisms or viruses such as hepatitis B and HIV.

Substances which are in contact with the skin or that otherwise enter the body can produce local effects at the point of contact and/or distant effects during the progress through the body. This has been categorized as:

1. Local – irritant to the skin, eyes or respiratory tract or allergic to the skin or respiratory tract and/or
2. Systemic – inherent toxicity and/or metabolite toxicity.

The hazard assessment and identification of risks to health can be further assisted by identifying the physical, biological, chemical, ergonomic or psychological causes.

Some clearer information regarding risk has been introduced by the Chemicals (Hazard Information and Packaging) Regulations 1993 which replaced the Classification, Packaging and Labelling of Dangerous Substances Regulations 1985 in September 1993. Substances which may be carcinogenic, mutagenic, or teratogenic are labelled with the toxic substances symbol – the skull and cross-bones. The definitions, with the accepted risk phrases, are as follows:

1. Carcinogenic – chemicals which may increase the incidence of cancer. These are further divided into categories 1 and 2 covering substances known to be carcinogenic to humans and are identified by the toxic substances symbol and R45 – the risk phrase which indicates 'may cause cancer'. Category 3 covers substances which

cause concern for humans. This category is used for substances where there is evidence from appropriate animal studies that the substance is carcinogenic but there is insufficient evidence to warrant a category 2 classification for humans. These substances will be identified by the harmful symbol (the black cross) and R40 – the risk phrase which indicates 'possible risk of irreversible effects'.

Substances which are carcinogenic only when inhaled are identified by the toxic substances symbol and R49 – the risk phrase 'may cause cancer by inhalation'.

2. Mutagenic – chemicals which may induce heritable genetic defects or increase their incidence.
3. Teratogenic – chemicals which may cause non-heritable birth defects in offspring of those exposed.
4. Substances dangerous for the environment are identified by a dead tree and a dead fish.

ASSESSMENT OF TOXIC HAZARDS

To make a preliminary assessment of the risks caused by toxic hazards it is essential to obtain some baseline information such as:

1. The name of the substance(s) and any synonyms.
2. A physical description of the chemical, e.g. particulate, gas, liquid, etc.
3. Identification of risks of exposure during handling or as a by-product of manufacture.
4. Exposure limits, if available.
5. Toxicological data including the route of entry into the body, the category of danger and risk, signs and symptoms.
6. Recommended handling procedures.
7. Recommended first aid and treatment.
8. Recommended personal protective equipment.

Information to support the hazard assessment will be supplied with the chemicals by the suppliers or manufacturers. The gathered information can then be evaluated by reference to the current edition of the HSE publication *Occupational Exposure Limits*. The lack of an exposure limit is not an indication of safety but a lack of data.

The Chemicals (Hazard Information and Packaging) Regulations 1993 (CHIP) are intended to protect people from the ill effects of dangerous chemicals by ensuring that hazards are correctly identified by using the 19 categories of danger and standard risk phrases; safety information should be supplied along with the chemicals and the packaging of chemical products must be suitable and secure.

The supplying of data sheets with the chemicals will make an assessment and self-protection easier, due to the 16 mandatory headings for CHIP Safety Data Sheets:

- Identification of the substance/preparation and the company
- Composition/information on ingredients
- Hazard identification
- First aid measures
- Fire-fighting measures
- Accidental release measures
- Handling and storage
- Exposure controls and personal protective equipment
- Physical and chemical properties
- Stability and reactivity
- Toxicological information
- Ecological information
- Disposal considerations
- Transport information
- Regulatory information
- Other information (training needs, data sources, etc.)

SOME DISEASES OF OCCUPATIONS

DISEASES OF THE RESPIRATORY SYSTEM

The lungs

The lungs are the first organ reached by inhaled substances.

Lung cancer is a common cancer. Cigarette smoking is the largest cause of non-occupational lung cancer. Information, and hopefully improved awareness and appreciation of the risks from exposure to carcinogens in some workplaces, has been increased with the introduction of CHIP.

Asthma is a very common disease and its importance in the workplace has recently been recognized as such. Occupational asthma is a reportable disease under RIDDOR and is a prescribed disease. Agents which are known to increase the risk of occupational asthma are designated in *Occupational Exposure Limits* by the note 'Sen' denoting the substance can cause sensitization. There is some debate about the increased risk of exposing atopics to sensitizing agents. Atopics are those who have a history of childhood asthma, eczema or hay fever, or people who show a positive skin reaction to skin prick testing with common allergens. They may have an increased risk of developing occupational asthma from exposure to enzymes, insects and platinum salts. The increasing incidence of childhood asthma will demand greater vigilance and strict control of environmental pollution in the workplace in the future.

Chronic respiratory disease can follow inhalation of substances which set up inflammation in the lungs which can eventually lead to fibrosis of the lung tissue. Some of the more common substances identified are: asbestos – asbestosis; cadmium – emphysema; coal dust – complicating simple pneumoconiosis; cobalt – hard metal disease; cotton dust – byssinosis; silica – silicosis; and talc – talcosis.

Extrinsic allergic alveolitis is an allergic response to an inhaled organic matter often a fungal protein from mouldy materials. The more common work groups at risk are: farmers – farmer's lung due to inhalation of fungi in mouldy hay; bird handlers – bird fancier's lung due to inhalation of the protein in dried bird droppings; mushroom worker's lung – due to inhalation of mushroom compost; cork producer's lung – suberosis caused by inhalation of mouldy cork; malt worker's lung due to inhalation of mouldy malt or barley; and cheese washer's lung due to inhalation of mouldy cheese.

The nose

Nasal cancer is uncommon in the general population. There are strong associations with exposure to nickel subsulphide in nickel refining, wood and leather dusts and the development of nasal cancer.

Rhinitis is a common complaint in the general population. Rhinitis can be a troublesome problem following exposure to dusts which are irritant, acid or alkaline and allergenic.

DISEASES OF THE LIVER

If absorption of a substance has taken place, the organs of metabolism and excretion – the liver and kidneys – can be challenged by the toxic substance or its metabolites. The liver, being the organ of detoxification of substances which are absorbed into the body, can be damaged even though it has a great capacity for regeneration. A wide range of agents encountered at work can have a primary effect on liver cells causing liver disease. Some substances which can damage or kill the liver cells are: acrylonitrile; alcohols; aliphatic chlorinated hydrocarbons (e.g. carbon tetrachloride, methyl chloride, tetrachloroethylene, trichloro- thane, vinyl chloride); aromatic nitro compounds (e.g. nitrobenzene, trinitrotoluene, etc.); phenol absorbed through the skin; selenium, yellow phosphorus, etc.

The liver is also at risk from infection leading to hepatitis. Two causative agents are leptospirosis icterhaemorrhagic – a risk to people involved in sewer work or exposed to water contaminated by the urine of infected rodents. This is also of concern to those participating in water sports. Health care workers are at risk from the range of hepatitis viruses – essentially blood borne.

Liver cancer can also occur from exposure to, for example, vinyl chloride monomer.

THE URINARY TRACT

The kidneys

Damage to the kidneys is often identified at routine health surveillance where routine urinalysis identifies protein in the urine. Substances such as cadmium and to a lesser extent mercury can lead to kidney disease.

The bladder

Cancer of the bladder can be caused by substances absorbed following exposure in the working environment as it is the organ in longest contact with the carcinogen. Some of the aromatic amines such as 4 aminodiphenyl; benzidene; and 1,2 naphthylamines are proven bladder carcinogens.

CENTRAL NERVOUS SYSTEM

The central nervous system can be affected by substances which cause anoxia. These substances can be divided into two simple categories of substances

1. Substances which are asphyxiants and replace oxygen in breathed air, such as methane and nitrogen.
2. Substances which prevent the red blood cells carrying oxygen, such as carbon monoxide.

The brain

The brain can be affected by high concentrations of substances such as chlorinated hydrocarbons, aliphatic hydrocarbons and aromatic hydrocarbons which have a narcotic effect and can lead to acute symptoms of drowsiness, inattention, mood swings and even death. The risks following exposure are increased due to the effect on employees exposed to the range of substances and involved in high risk occupations such as driving and machine operation.

THE CARDIOVASCULAR SYSTEM

Coronary artery disease is a common problem in the population generally. In the work context there are some substances, such as carbon disulphide, which at sufficient levels are recognized to cause coronary artery disease. The manufacture of nitrates such as glycol denigrate and nitro-glycerine is linked with some sudden deaths due to heart failure. This has occurred particularly after periods of absence from exposure.

Inhalation of chlorinated and fluorinated hydrocarbons can cause irregularities of the heart beat and again, in extreme cases, has led to sudden death.

THE SKIN

Primary contact dermatitis

Primary contact dermatitis is the most common type of dermatitis. In 1992 the various schemes reported an incidence of 411 cases – DSS II; two cases of chrome ulceration, folliculitis and acne – RIDDOR; and 2636 cases – EPIDERM (HSC Annual Report, 1992/93).

For risk assessment purposes primary contact dermatitis can be considered thus:

1. Contact with strong acids and alkalines will cause skin irritation in everyone exposed. The response depends on the strength of the substance and the length of time in contact with the skin. Concentrated sulphuric acid will cause a response in a few seconds. Soap and water may take several days before they cause a clinically noticeable change.
2. Contact with the primary skin irritants will cause a reaction in the majority of people after repeated exposure. The substances involved have specific effects on the unprotected skin, making it more vulnerable to further damage following repeated and regular contact, e.g. solvents. The practice of some employees of using non-skin preparations such as turpentine, petrol, etc. for skin cleansing adds to the risks of developing primary irritant contact dermatitis. Soluble oils, some paints and plant products also lead to skin degreasing.

The prevention of contact dermatitis due to contact with primary irritants is basically to select safer substances for use, the control of the dilution of substances used, a high level of personal hygiene and the selection and use of suitable hand cleansers. The thorough drying of the hands after washing, the application of skin conditioning creams at the end of the working day and easy access to professional advice providing adequate treatment can all make a positive contribution.

The diagnosis of primary contact dermatitis is based on the occupational history, site of lesions and the progress of the condition. As with a number of occupational diseases the reaction and symptoms tend to subside over the weekends and during holidays only to reccur on return to work. If the complaint does not improve after removal from work exposure for long periods then another source of contact should be considered. The use of a growing range of chemicals in the home, the pursuit of hobbies or additional employment may have to be explored and considered.

The site of the lesions may assist in the diagnosis, such as the glove distribution. The general response is usually seen on exposed skin surfaces such as the hands, forearms, wrists and cubital fossa which are in direct contact with the known or suspected agent. Gases, fumes and vapours can cause an effect on areas other than the hands and arms, such as the neck, face and chest due to the tendency of gases, fumes and vapours to rise and move with the air currents. Smoke detector tubes or a Tyndall Beam can assist in making the movement visible.

Allergic contact dermatitis

Allergic contact dermatitis is attributed to substances with a molecular weight of 150 to 300 which penetrate the skin and set up an allergic response. The period of time between exposure and development of the allergic reaction can be several years after initial contact. Once the allergic reaction has been established contact with the identified sensitizer must be avoided. On re-exposure the reaction can reccur after a short delay. Employees developing allergic contact dermatitis may have to be removed from further exposure or at the very least they must ensure that they do not have direct skin contact with the causative substance. Some of the more common categories of substances which can cause skin allergy are aniline derivatives such as TNT; antibiotics such as penicillin and the tetracyclines; dyes used in inks and cosmetics (lanolin which is common in hand conditioners and some soaps); metals such as chromate, nickel and cobalt; resins such as epoxy and formaldehyde resins, vinyl and acrylics; rubber accelerators, vulcanizers and antioxidants; plants such as primula, chrysanthemums and tulips; and trees such as West African mahogany and the red cedar.

The list of substances causing skin allergy is long and it is often difficult to establish the real cause of the skin reaction. The standard battery of patch testing may have to be completed to identify the specific agent.

Non-dermatitic causes of skin diseases

Ultraviolet light

The dangers of continued and excessive exposure to ultraviolet light (UVL) have been highlighted by the increasing number of new cases of melanoma. People working out of doors in occupations such as construction and farming are at an increasing risk. The relatively common practice of outdoor workers of stripping to the waist on hot sunny days to obtain a deep tan will increase their risk of developing melanoma and is to be avoided. Other skin effects of overexposure to ultraviolet light are premature ageing of the skin, pigmentation, acute burns, phototoxic reactions and photosensitive reactions due to some drugs and chrome.

The reduction of the risk to outdoor workers can be achieved by ensuring they cover exposed skin surfaces and use creams and lotions which contain an ultraviolet blocker on all exposed skin surfaces. Eyes must also be protected by the wearing of dark glasses.

Infra-red radiation

Exposure to infra-red (IR) can cause heat stress and burns. The risks occur in occupations which expose the worker to high levels of thermal energy such as occupations in glass blowing and the metal industries. Glass workers' cataracts have occurred following long exposure to the white-hot surfaces of the glass. The skin reactions to IR radiation are vasodilatation and following repeated exposure, skin pigmentation and burns.

Skin infections

Skin infections are common in some occupations where animals and organic matter are handled. Workers who have their hands in water for long periods of time such as in the food industry and the health care sector have an increased risk of skin infection, particularly paronychia.

Skin cancers

Skin cancers tend to be slow to develop and when chemicals are involved can develop following heavy and prolonged contact. Some of the more common physical causes are exposure to ultraviolet light and ionizing radiation. Some of the chemicals which can cause skin cancers are polycyclic aromatic hydrocarbons such as tar, mineral oils, pitch and soot.

The prognosis for skin cancer tends to be better than for many other types of cancer as there is usually earlier recognition and consequently earlier treatment.

MUSCULO-SKELETAL INJURIES

Musculo-skeletal injuries in employment are rarely caused by a single sudden accident or injury but by a series of repeated microtrauma leading to cumulative injury. The high incidence of musculo-skeletal problems in the working population, ages 18 to 64, is higher than in any other group of people. The onset of disability and pain can be slow and as a consequence dismissed by the sufferer until the symptoms become persistent and chronic. The preventive theory relates to the identification through risk assessment of activities or occupations which require force plus repetitive activity plus static or anatomically awkward positions and with insufficient recovery times.

WORK RELATED UPPER LIMB DISORDERS

The debate as to whether the results of microtrauma are regarded as accidents or are an example of the disease process is still to be clarified for reporting and investigation purposes. Conditions under the UK description of Work Related Upper Limb Disorder (WRULD) are not required to be reported under RIDDOR. In 1992/93 there were reported through the DSS II schemes 649 cases of tenosynovitis, 317 cases of beat conditions and 52 cases of upper limb cramp (HSC Annual Report, 1992/93). These conditions are only prescribed diseases for specified occupations or activities.

The Management of Health and Safety at Work Regulations 1992, the Health and Safety (Display Screen Equipment) Regulations 1992 (1992a) and the Manual Handling Operations Regulations 1992 (1992b) require the employer to complete risk assessments to identify the activities or environmental conditions which could lead to injury, and there is a general requirement to reduce the identified risks as far as practicable.

WRULD relates to the collection of chronic musculo-skeletal injuries caused by some aspect of repetitive work. Unlike sudden sprains and strains there are few, if any, immediately identifiable causes or events. The early symptoms can be similar to those experienced following a sprain such as localized pain, swelling and loss of function.

Disorders of tendons

Tendon disorders often occur at or near the joints where the tendon rubs nearby ligaments and bones. The most frequent complaint relates to a dull ache over the tendon, discomfort with specific movements, and tenderness to touch. There is seldom noticeable redness or local heat and recovery is usually slow. The condition may easily become chronic if the cause is not eliminated.

Tendonitis is tendon inflammation which can occur when a muscle/tendon group is repeatedly tensed. With continuous exertion, some of the tendon fibres can actually fray or tear apart. The tendon becomes thickened, bumpy and irregular. Without rest and sufficient time for the tissues to heal, the tendon may be permanently damaged.

Disorders of sheathed tendons

Tenosynovitis is a general term for a repetitive induced tendon injury involving the synovial sheath. With continuous repetitive actions, the sheath produces excessive amounts of synovial fluid. The synovial fluid accumulates in the tendon sheath which becomes swollen and painful. If the tendon surface becomes rough, and if the sheath becomes inflamed and continues to press on the tendon, stenosing tenosynovitis may occur. For example, when the tendon sheath of a finger is sufficiently swollen to lock the tendon in the sheath, movement of the affected finger causes a jerking movement commonly referred to as 'trigger finger'. The palm side of the finger is the usual site for the trigger finger response.

De Quervain's Contracture can be caused by excessive friction between the two thumb tendons and their common sheath. Repetitive activities lead to friction and subsequent abnormal thickening of the fibrous sheath resulting in constriction of the tendons.

Ganglions, often on the wrist(s), are cysts which occur when the effected sheath swells up with synovial fluid and causes a bump under the skin. In the past ganglions were called 'Bible bumps' as the popular treatment was to use the Bible, or similar heavy object, to hit the swelling sharply on the wrist to rupture the ganglion.

Disorders of unsheathed tendons

If unsheathed tendons, such as are found in the elbow and shoulder joints, are injured the area may eventually calcify. When strained or over used, the tendons become irritated and pain is radiated from the elbow down to the forearm, which is referred to as lateral epicondylitis. Common activities that lead to the condition are associated with impact or jerky throwing motions. The resulting condition is commonly referred to as 'tennis elbow' or 'frozen shoulder'.

Neurovascular disorders

Some WRULDs involve both the nerves and adjacent blood vessels, and are referred to as thoracic outlet syndrome. This is a general term describing compression of the nerves and blood vessels between the neck and shoulder which is common in activities such as keyboard work. The sufferer may complain of symptoms such as numbness in the fingers of the hand, or pins and needles, or may describe the sensation of the arm feeling as though it is 'going to sleep'. On examination the pulse at the wrist may be weakened.

REGULATION AND HEALTH SURVEILLANCE

The current provision of heatlh surveillance in the UK is changing. Initially health surveillance was implemented:

1. to meet regulatory requirements;
2. to provide pre-employment health surveillance programmes (in support of the human resources function);
3. to reduce the impact of claims for compensation;
4. to support the termination of employment on grounds of ill health;
5. to advise on the fitness of employees to return to work following absence attributed to ill health.

The Management of Health and Safety at Work Regulations 1992 now require the employer to complete risk assessment and to provide appropriate health surveillance. This is a much wider requirement linked to the risks of the organization and the concept of self-regulation.

HEALTH SURVEILLANCE RECORDS

There is a large amount of duplication of health surveillance programmes. This risk of duplication of health surveillance appears to be unlikely to be changed. For example, the Health and Safety (Display Screen Equipment) Regulations 1992, regulation 5 requires eyes and eyesight tests to be provided on request to defined users of the display screen equipment. This can result in the mobile workforce being examined several times in a short timespan as there is little referral or sharing of information or records between companies.

If directed research and subsequent strategies for the prevention of occupational disease are to be progressed then access to factual practical information is essential. For 50% of the working population there are health surveillance records held by employing organizations. For employees working under the health surveillance programmes required by the Control of Substances Hazardous to Health Regulations 1988 and related amendments there may be the results of environmental and biological monitoring. Many organizations implement specific projects directed to their own unique problems. A large amount of valuable information and data has been produced but little of it is available to other interested parties.

When a company closes, the records are often destroyed. The HSE will not take them; the professional advisory bodies have a concern regarding confidentiality but provide little practical advice in respect of the retention of records. The end result is that 50% of the workforce through their working life have health examinations which are used by their current employer. The real value of a life occupational record, showing exposures, type of work, preventive strategies, results of biological monitoring and environmental exposure is lost due to the very nature of the legislation, the fragmented control of records and the personnel bias of a high proportion of health surveillance programmes. This retained health surveillance data is often used by employers in cases of litigation. But surely the real benefit to society is the reduction of the risk and incidence of occupational disease. The employee's previous exposure is key to this objective.

As referred to earlier, GPs and consultants diagnose more cases of occupational disease than are reported to the HSE. A large proportion of the population believe they are suffering work related disease and self refer. The records made by the GP are available to the patient under the Access to Medical Reports Act 1988. The GP records tend to be made over a long period of time and are extensive as there is little opportunity for editing by the patient. Is the time right to explore a change of direction of occupational health services? Or as a minimum, to consider the value and introduction of worker held health surveillance records?

MANAGEMENT ISSUES

In the 1970s the Robens report set in train the shift from prescriptive regulations towards the broader obligations of the Health and Safety at Work etc. Act 1974 and the concept of self-regulation.

Research programmes completed by the Health and Safety Executive's Accident Prevention Advisory Unit (APAU) in the 1980s found that 70% to 75% of accidents were due to management failures (HSE, 1985). In successive Health and Safety Commission (HSC) reports references were made to high standards of managerial control as key to high standards of occupational health and safety (Health and Safety Commission Annual Report, 1986/87). It was also suggested that many organizations which could demonstrate high standards of general business management could also demonstrate a commitment to the notion of self-regulation. The emerging definition of self-regulation is not just self-enforcement of the rules and regulations made by outsiders, but involves the purposeful creation and maintenance of specific tailor-made standards and controls consistent with the risks inherent in the employer's undertaking.

In 1987/88 it was evident that the HSC was undertaking a review of the detail of health and safety legislation which was and is perceived as a burden by some employers. The work of reform and simplification is in line with the government's aim to reduce the large amount of specific and often prescriptive out of date legislation which the regulatory bodies have been working to and which sometimes makes it difficult for enterprises to prosper. This work is continuing today amid fears of reduction of the protection that legislation and enforcement provides for the employees working in establishments with health professionals. It is of greater concern to the 50% who do not work for these caring employers.

The importance of managing health and safety is reflected in the publication by HSE (1991) of *Successful Health and Safety Management*. The concept of managing and auditing health and safety is slowly gaining momentum. The philosophy is based on the concept that well-managed organizations are safe organizations. A great deal of the guidance on managing health and safety as any other function is based on the principles of Total Quality Management (TQM). TQM can be defined as philosophies and company practices that aim to harness the human and material resources of an organization in the most effective way to achieve the objectives of the organization. In BS 7850 this traditional view of TQM is indicated as a philosophy which recognizes that business objectives, customer satisfaction, environmental considerations, and health and safety are interdependent. The philosophy of TQM can be applied to any organization. Is this a concept that can be promoted to reduce the high incidence of occupational disease?

The challenge for those health professionals working to reduce the incidence of occupational disease may well be to recognize the merits of working as facilitators, that is, as health professionals continuing to work to enable managers to establish adequate policies, appropriate organization for the implementation of such policies and accountability at the highest level. The objective is for managers to manage the reduction of the incidence of occupational ill health. The next management steps are to measure the effectiveness of the systems through the collection of data and the implementation of monitoring and auditing programmes. For the health professionals it will mean moving away from the pure medical model to a risk management model.

Health professionals and the government must not ignore the half of the workforce in the UK that does not have the benefit of working for an employer who provides professional health care. It can be argued that it is this population who are at most risk.

REFERENCES

British Standards Institution BS 7850: Part 1: 1992.
Central Statistical Office (1987) *Annual Abstract of Statistics*, Central Statistical Office, London.
Charley, I.H. (1954) *The Birth of Industrial Nursing*, Baillière Tindall, London, UK.
Chemicals (Hazard Information and Packaging) Regulations 1993 (Statutory Instrument 1993 No. 1746), HMSO, London, UK.
Control of Asbestos at Work Regulations 1987 (Statutory Instrument 1987, No. 2115), HMSO, London, UK.
Department of Health (1991) *The Health of the Nation* (Cm 1523), HMSO, London, UK.
Doll, R. and Peto, J. (1985) *Effects on health of exposure to asbestos*, HSE Books, Sudbury, UK.
Health and Safety Commission (1993) Control of Substances Hazardous to Health and Control of Carcinogenic Substances. Control of Substances Hazardous to Health Regulations 1988. Approved Codes of Practice. 4th edn. (*L5 Series*) HSE Books, Sudbury, UK.
Health and Safety Commission Annual Report 1986/87. HSE Books, Sudbury, UK.
Health and Safety Commission Annual Report 1990/91. HSE Books, Sudbury, UK.
Health and Safety Commission Annual Report 1992/93. HSE Books, Sudbury, UK.
Health and Safety Commission Annual Report 1992/93 Statistical Supplement. HSE Books, Sudbury, UK.
Health and Safety Commission Plan of work for 1992/93 and beyond. HSE Books, Sudbury, UK.
Health and Safety Executive (1985) Monitoring Safety: an outline report on occupational safety and health by the Accident Advisory Unit. *HSE Occasional Paper 9*, HSE Books, Sudbury, UK.
Health and Safety Executive (1992a) Display Screen Equipment Work. Health and Safety (Display Screen Equipment) Regulations 1992. Guidance on Regulations L26. HSE Books, Sudbury, UK.
Health and Safety Executive (1992b) Manual Handling. Manual Handling Operations Regulations 1992. Guidance on Regulations L23. HSE Books, Sudbury, UK.
Health and Safety Executive (annual) *Occupational Exposure Limits*. HSE Books, Sudbury, UK.

Health and Safety Executive (1991) *Successful health and safety management*. (HS(G) 65), HSE Books, Sudbury, UK.

Rosen, G. (1943) *The History of Miners' Diseases: a medical and social interpretation*, Schuman, New York, USA.

Schilling, R.S.F. (ed.) (1981) *Occupational Health Practice*, Butterworths & Co. (Publishers) Ltd, London, UK.

Toxicology in the workplace

6

Steve Fairhurst

INTRODUCTION

Toxicology is the study of the adverse effects of substances on biological systems and the assessment of the likelihood that such effects will occur in specified circumstances. This involves two separable but related activities: the identification of the hazardous properties of chemicals (their inherent potential to cause harm) and assessment of the likelihood that those hazardous properties will be expressed under defined exposure conditions (i.e. the risk involved in particular circumstances). The nature of the work covers a wide spectrum, ranging from attempts to predict the effects of substances based on chemical structure and physicochemical properties, through a wide range of experimental possibilities, to observations in humans and epidemiological findings. All adverse health effects arising from the chemical nature of a substance are manifestations of 'toxicity' and all substances have some toxicological properties. Hence, toxicology in relation to the workplace necessitates consideration of any of the enormous number of chemical substances now in commercial use and the potential impact of those substances on people at work. The nature of the toxicology task should be to acquire relevant data, critically assess its value and significance, and assemble the most detailed and accurate picture possible of the hazards and risks to health posed by the substance and situation. This work should bring about important interactions between toxicology and other disciplines – occupational medicine, epidemiology and occupational hygiene – the collective aim being to develop a sound scientific and technical basis for good health standards and control measures in the workplace.

Some toxicological issues are simple and obvious, requiring no more than ordinary common sense to resolve. For example, one does not need to be the toxicology equivalent of a rocket scientist to realize that highly concentrated, strong acids on the skin will burn and that protective measures are indicated to limit the risk of skin damage in use. However, many issues are considerably more complex, requiring well-developed specialist skills if they are to be thoroughly addressed. This chapter is written from within a regulatory authority and from the standpoint of a specialist group with considerable toxicological expertise. Obviously the UK Health and Safety Executive (HSE) is by no means unique in this respect; there are quite a few big fish in the pond. Nonetheless, clearly there are also many people throughout industry in the UK and elsewhere who are faced with workplace regulatory issues involving toxicology and who do not have such specialist resources readily available. Hence it should be acknowledged from the start that, in places, what follows might appear somewhat idealistic. Without making an apology for this, it must be stressed that the intention here is not to lecture or be prescriptive, nor to attempt to present in this chapter official regulatory authority policy in this area. The intention is simply to present a perspective and to raise a range of issues for consideration.

BACKGROUND

The regulatory framework in the UK and other countries has for some time contained a general requirement to protect the health of the workforce against the potential threats offered by chemical substances. Nevertheless, it is true to say that the enormous and rapid expansion in the number of chemical substances in the occupational environment in the last few decades has taken place largely in the absence of regulatory schemes specifically requiring the gathering and critical assessment of detailed and comprehensive toxicological data. The result is that substances have been examined *ad hoc* in a very patchy pattern. A minority of substances have been well investigated, unfortunately sometimes because health effects in humans had already become evident. However, most substances of interest in relation to occupational exposure do not have extensive, detailed toxicological data on them, and many have not been investigated at all.

There has been an attitude of 'no news is good news', meaning by this that the absence of reports of health effects directly observed in worker populations has been taken as assurance that there is no problem. Although there is some justification for this view, one has to ask whether anyone has actually properly looked for any potential effects in populations exposed to the chemical of interest and, even if someone has been looking, whether or not some of the potential effects for particular substances would have been revealed from the nature of the investigation.

Overall, in terms of thoroughness and reliability, the toxicology scene in relation to industrial chemicals and occupational exposure has lagged behind that of certain other classes of chemical, such as pharmaceuticals. However, marked changes in the regulatory aspect of occupational toxicology have occurred in recent years. In general, there is now a more questioning, challenging attitude towards established positions. This makes it essential that stances adopted in relation to chemical control are robust; this requires the toxicology element to be based on clear and thoroughly documented critical appraisal of data obtained directly from identified original sources. Documentation explaining in detail the basis for a regulatory position is expected to be readily available for scrutiny and must be of a quality to withstand such examination.

There are also now powerful regulatory programmes which entail detailed assessment of the toxicology of substances and impinge on workplace control. From a UK perspective these programmes are both national and international in nature, with the international aspect growing ever larger and more significant. Some of these programmes are strictly statutory in nature, such as the EU '7th Amendment' (EEC, 1992), which has been implemented in the UK by the Notification of New Substances Regulations 1993 (NONS, 1993) and the Existing Substances Regulation (EEC, 1993a). Others are non-statutory but nevertheless highly influential, such as the OECD High Production Volume chemicals programme and the IPCS (International Programme on Chemical Safety) initiative to produce Environmental Health Criteria documents.

The net result of these developments is that the current climate in occupational regulatory toxicology demands high quality work, with clearly explained and documented positions based on full awareness and critical evaluation of original data.

GENERAL PRINCIPLES

Toxicology can be divided into two general areas, those of toxicokinetics (what the body does with the substance) and toxicodynamics (what the substance does to the body). Toxicokinetics involves exploration of:

- absorption of the substance (extent and rate) across the respiratory and gastrointestinal tracts and skin;
- distribution of the substance and/or its metabolites around the body;
- metabolism, i.e. the site(s), rate(s) and extent(s) of conversion of the substance to other chemical entities and the nature of the metabolites thus formed;

• excretion (extent, rate, route) from the body.

Toxicokinetic information can be invaluable in developing a full appreciation of the toxicity of a chemical. Several issues can be greatly clarified by such data. For instance, knowledge of the extent of absorption and pattern of distribution via particular exposure routes can be influential in deciding on which toxicity endpoints might merit further exploration. At its most sophisticated, toxicokinetic studies have helped enormously in our understanding of the toxicological properties of substances and the predictivity for humans of toxicity data obtained in particular experimental models, e.g. for dichloromethane (ECETOC, 1987).

Toxicodynamics, or 'toxicity', is conventionally sub-divided into:

• acute toxicity, i.e. the systemic consequences of single exposure;
• irritation/corrosivity towards the skin and eyes, resulting from surface contact with the substance;
• sensitization, both skin and respiratory;
• repeated dose toxicity, i.e. the consequences (excluding those effects covered by other categories in this list) of repeated exposure to the substance.
• mutagenicity, or genotoxicity;
• carcinogenicity;
• effects on reproduction:
   – fertility effects
   – developmental effects.

The occupational environment holds several exposure possibilities – single exposure under controlled (i.e. intended) conditions, single exposure under uncontrolled (i.e. accidental) conditions, occasional but repeated exposure, regular daily exposure under controlled conditions, and combinations of these. Exposure can also occur via more than one route. This means that for toxicology in an occupational exposure context, the entire range of toxicodynamic issues needs to be considered, and each in relation to the potential route(s) of exposure to the substance of interest.

ROUTES OF EXPOSURE

The two modes of exposure of primary concern in the workplace are inhalation of the airborne substance and surface (skin, eyes) contact with the substance. This can immediately pose some problems where one is seeking to predict the relevant hazards and the risks to health in an occupational context from an experimental animal database, where studies are often conducted with oral administration as the chosen

dosing route; data may also be available from studies involving par-
enteral injection.

If one is considering internal, systemic effects, such as liver damage
or central nervous system depression, then extrapolation from the
findings of studies involving non-occupational routes of exposure is
often possible, although problematic. One has to have some appreciation of the similarities and differences in the toxicokinetics of the
substance (i.e. the rate and extent of absorption and the manner in
which it is handled by the body once inside) between the exposure
route used and the exposure route of interest.

If one is considering local effects at the initial site of contact, then
route-to-route extrapolation is often very much more difficult, if not
impossible, in terms of dose-response relationships. For example, a
substance of moderately strong acidity may exert relatively minor effects
from its pH if ingested. However, the consequences of inhalation
through the impact of the acidity in the airway linings of the respiratory
tract could be very different and more serious. Similarly, repeated
ingestion of high doses of a poorly soluble solid may well have no
health consequences, the substance simply passing through the
gastrointestinal tract and out with the faeces; a comparable dose inhaled
into the lungs could give rise to severe dust reactions.

In general, if one is concerned with occupational exposure scenarios
it is clearly preferable, and sometimes essential, to deal with data
relating to exposure via occupationally relevant routes. The frequent
absence of such information, particularly the paucity of inhalation
exposure data for many substances, poses an interesting problem for
both regulatory authorities and industry in the occupational toxicology
field.

TYPES OF EFFECT

A wide variety of toxicological effects could conceivably arise as a result
of occupational exposure to a substance. Possibilities to be borne in
mind are shown in Table 6.1.

Interest surrounding specified endpoints could be in relation to a
single exposure situation, or may require repeated exposure, perhaps
over a prolonged period, or could be a feature of both exposure
regimes.

When faced with a chemical substance and concerns regarding
occupational exposure, consideration must be given to the full range of
issues raised above. Information relating to all aspects of the toxicological picture must be sought. Such information can take the form of
data obtained from investigations or observations involving precisely
the exposure situation and toxicological endpoint of interest. However,

Table 6.1 Toxicological effects of occupational exposure to substances

Nature of exposure	Local effects (site of contact)	Systemic effects
Inhalation	**Respiratory tract** Sensory irritation, i.e. nerve stimulation. Direct tissue damage. Respiratory sensitization. Inflammatory effects of particles. Mutagenicity; carcinogenicity.	Internal effects on organs and tissues following absorption. Consequences of transport of substances to gastrointestinal tract via mucociliary escalator and swallowing.
Skin contact	**Skin (eye)** Irritation (nerve stimulation, tissue inflammation). Corrosion. Skin sensitization. Mutagenicity; carcinogenicity.	Internal effects on organs and tissues following absorption. Consequences of manual transfer to oro-nasal cavities.

often such data are not available for a particular substance, necessitating an attempt to predict the position with respect to the situation of interest, from other information available on that substance and its analogues. Reliable predictions are sometimes, but by no means always, possible to make and sometimes acquisition of further data by way of experimental study or human observations may appear to be the best (possibly only?) way forward.

An essential aspect of occupational toxicology should be to set out what is not known (or readily predictable) about the hazardous properties and risks to health posed by the substance, as well as what is known (or readily predictable), and the degree of confidence/uncertainty one has in the accuracy and completeness of the toxicology picture presented. Unfortunately, all too often these points are not addressed.

SOURCES OF TOXICOLOGICAL INFORMATION

Within the occupational health and hygiene profession there has been a heavy reliance on what might be called 'classical' textbook sources of toxicological information. Publications such as Sax and Lewis' *Dangerous Properties of Industrial Materials* (Sax and Lavis, 1989) and Patty's *Industrial Hygiene and Toxicology* (Patty, 1963) have often been the first and only port of call. Latterly several computerized databases in a similar vein have also been developed. Such sources have been and will continue to be extremely helpful as brief general synopses of the known properties of some substances. They are readily at hand and the convenience and attraction of their use is obvious.

The question is whether or not the use of such sources alone represents a sufficiently rigorous approach to a toxicology issue. One obvious problem is that these sources do not cover all substances. Also, where a substance is covered, there can on occasion be problems concerning the identification of the original source and underpinning evidence for some of the statements made. The examples below are of statements made in such sources which we in HSE's Toxicology Unit have found impossible to verify from an exhaustive search of the primary literature on the substance in question. Furthermore, there is a tendency in such abbreviated presentations not to make clear what is not known (i.e. where there are no data) for the substance in question. One should always keep firmly in mind the degree to which the information source being used meets requirements, in terms of being up to date and thorough, and whether or not it incorporates the important feature of critical appraisal of the data being presented. In relation to this last point, toxicology is much more than a simple act of locating and passing on information. To properly address regulatory requirements involving occupational toxicology considerations, such as classification and labelling, safety data sheets, workplace risk assessments and occupational exposure limits, one needs to consider the full range of issues involved to ä considerably greater depth than that afforded by the kind of secondary sources discussed above. Obviously to recipients of safety data sheets and labelled substances, these regulatory features themselves should represent important sources of toxicological information.

UNVERIFIABLE TOXICOLOGICAL STATEMENTS FROM THE SECONDARY LITERATURE

- Patty's *Industrial Hygiene and Toxicology*, 2nd edn, vol. II, p. 1211 reports that exposure to 300 ppm cyclohexane is 'somewhat irritating to the eyes and mucous membranes' (Patty, 1963).
- Elkins' *The Chemistry of Industrial Toxicology*, 2nd edn, p. 121 reports that workers exposed to 100 ppm methyl isobutyl ketone 'complained of headache and nausea' (Elkins, 1959).

Neither of these statements gives a reference pointing to an original source of data to substantiate the claim, nor could such a reference be found elsewhere in the literature.

The opposite end of the spectrum involves a detailed critical assessment by toxicology specialists of all the original data available on a substance, obtained from primary sources. This very rigorous approach is adopted by the relevant regulatory authority in the UK (HSE) and in certain other countries, by some major chemicals companies and industry associations and by international programmes such as the International Programme on Chemical Safety (IPCS) when dealing with substances and issues of high priority and interest. It is aimed at ensuring thoroughness and reliability in the toxicological assessment produced, but also requires a substantial resource input in terms of time, effort and expertise. Many of these reviewing activities result in the production of published documents which set out in considerable detail the toxicology of the substances addressed. Examples are the IPCS Environmental Health Criteria documents, the Criteria Documents for establishing occupational exposure limits produced by several European countries (e.g. the UK, The Netherlands, Sweden) and the European Chemical Industry Ecology and Toxicology Centre (ECETOC) Technical Reports. Such documents are usually of high quality and can provide a reliable picture of the toxicology of individual substances.

These publications present a very important potential source of information, especially for those faced with a need for a toxicological assessment but without the resources and time available to review the substance themselves. Also, moves are now taking place, under the auspices of institutions/programmes such as IPCS and European Union Health and Safety Directorate (CEC DG V), to create a situation whereby organizations producing such detailed critical reviews follow common principles and produce a document of specific quality and format. By such means, all such reviews would contribute to an internationally available pool of reliable toxicological assessments and duplication of effort by several different organizations each reviewing the same substance could be avoided.

In the HSE, detailed assessments of this type have been produced for regulatory outcomes such as the setting of occupational exposure limits or the establishment of an agreed classification and labelling position. Other regulatory authority documentation surrounding these programmes such as the Approved List (HSC, 1993), derived from Annexe I of the EEC Directive on Classification, Packaging and Labelling of Dangerous Substances (EEC, 1967) and EH 64 (HSE, 1993a) represents another valuable source of brief toxicological information. Again, other countries engaged in such regulatory work also produce similar material.

HAZARD AND RISK

No discussion of occupational toxicology would be complete without making a big issue of the terms 'hazard' and 'risk'. It is necessary to clarify meanings because some elements of occupational regulatory toxicology focus on identification of hazard, whereas others focus on assessment of risk and some programmes require both areas to be addressed. Understanding this is essential.

Things ought to be quite straightforward. In the regulatory toxicology context, hazard refers to the intrinsic toxicological properties of a substance, i.e. the effects it is capable of producing when administered by various routes of exposure. Risk refers to the likelihood of the toxicological properties being expressed under specified exposure conditions. The two can be linked together by attempting to construct a dose – response relationship for the substance and effect(s) and then relating to this relationship a known or predicted level of exposure. Ambiguity or confusion surrounding hazard and risk arises either because the two terms are used loosely and almost interchangeably, or because one or the other term is used when neither is appropriate.

Classification and labelling of substances and preparations under the relevant EU Directives and Amendments (EEC, 1967; EEC, 1988) and in UK terms the Chemicals (Hazard Information and Packaging) Regulations 1993 (CHIP, 1993), deal exclusively with the province of hazard identification. Establishment of suitable occupational exposure limits is a risk assessment issue. The toxicological testing and data evaluation procedures contained within the EU 7th Amendment (UK Notification of New Substances Regulations) and Existing Substances Regulation (ESR) encompass both hazard identification and risk assessment as defined procedural steps (EEC, 1992; EEC, 1993a).

HAZARD IDENTIFICATION, CLASSIFICATION AND LABELLING

Identification of the hazardous properties, i.e. the intrinsic toxicological features, of a substance is the starting point for the toxicologist in building up a picture of the potential health impact of and the appropriate regulatory measures to apply to a substance. Hazard identification is the endpoint for much of the standard regulatory toxicity testing performed on substances (some tests also yield dose – response information). Hazard identification is also the philosophy underlying EU classification and labelling, one of the key features of the overall regulatory strategy to control industrial chemicals. In this respect it is unfortunate that in relation to one critical element of the EU classification and labelling system, the phrases used to indicate toxicological properties are erroneously termed 'risk' phrases. Obviously they describe hazard, not risk.

For the supply of chemicals to be used in workplaces (and elsewhere) there is a regulatory requirement to classify and label substances, and formulations, in accordance with the EU-wide system described in EU Directives (with Amendments) on the Classification and Labelling of Dangerous Substances and Preparations and the Annexes thereof (EEC, 1967; EEC, 1988). In the UK this system is implemented through the Chemicals (Hazard Identification and Packaging) Regulations (CHIP, 1993).

The system requires that identified hazardous toxicological properties, from whatever test situation used or observations made, are considered in terms of their relevance to human health and the classification and labelling ultimately derived should reflect this relevance. All the data available on a chemical, including both experimental animal and human findings, need to be taken into account. For some issues, such as acute toxicity or skin irritation, the criteria are relatively straightforward and easy to apply. In other areas such as carcinogenicity or reproductive toxicity things can get somewhat more tricky, with much greater scope and need for careful consideration and interpretation of the findings of both experimental studies and epidemiological findings.

NEW SUBSTANCES

Substances first introduced into the EU market after September 1981, and hence not listed in the European Inventory of Existing Commercial Chemical Substances (EINECS), are subject to the notification requirements of the 7th Amendment; in the UK this programme is implemented via the Notification of New Substances Regulations 1993 (EEC, 1992; NONS, 1993). Among other things this scheme requires the generation, by the manufacturer or importer, of a package of toxicity tests on the 'new substance' in question and the submission of full reports of such tests to the appropriate regulatory authority in one of the member states, to be assessed for conformity with requirements and interpretation of the findings. One of the principal regulatory outcomes is the determination of the appropriate classification and labelling for the substance.

The EU classification and labelling scheme, as it relates to the use of experimental animal findings, is geared to accommodate most easily the results of tests conducted to current internationally recognized standard OECD guidelines. As testing of new substances must be performed in accordance with these methods, the results thereby generated should readily slot into the classification and labelling criteria. Notification to and acceptance by the regulatory authority is an essential pre-marketing requirement for new substances. Therefore, although the extent of toxicity testing is limited at the initial stage, nevertheless the principle is that new substances and preparations containing them being supplied to workplaces (and elsewhere) arrive for the first time with some of their potential toxicological endpoints having already been explored and, where indicated by the findings, some of the hazardous properties shown on the label.

As the quantity of a new substance on the market increases, then consideration is given to more extensive testing embracing a wider range of potential endpoints and greater depth of detail. The results of earlier tests are an influential factor in the approach taken to further toxicity testing. Again the EU classification and labelling criteria are applied to the results of such testing to update the position regarding hazard identification. Therefore the picture is one of classification and labelling indicating the hazardous properties of a new substance which have shown up in the standard experimental studies required to be performed on such substances, with such testing being gradually built up in a structured manner.

EXISTING SUBSTANCES

The respective situation for existing (i.e. EINECS-listed) substances is partly the same, partly quite different. It is the same in the sense that the same general EU classification and labelling system and criteria apply. It is different in that there has been no associated requirement to generate toxicity data to which the classification and labelling criteria can be applied.

Hence the supplier (and the regulator) must make use of whatever information is available in relation to the toxicological properties of the substance in question. The quantity and quality of this information will vary enormously for different substances, as indicated earlier. The obligation is with the supplier to apply the classification and labelling criteria in the most appropriate manner to any substance or preparation, across the whole range of toxicological endpoints.

The toxicological issues involved can become quite complex and require considerable expertise to arrive at the appropriate solution. An example is given on pages 129–30. It features three substances, each of which is clearly carcinogenic in rodents by an administration route relevant to human exposure. However, the appropriate EU carcinogenicity classification for each is different, illustrating the complexity of toxicological consideration that needs to be applied in some circumstances.

EU CARCINOGENICITY CLASSIFICATION

These three chemicals need to be considered in relation to their EU classification for carcinogenicity. The following information is available from animal and *in vitro* test systems; there are no useful human data in relation to this endpoint.

Substance A

Rats and mice exposed to 400 ppm by inhalation for two years. Increased malignant tumours in the nasal cavity in both species.

Substance B

Rats and mice exposed orally to 600–1200 ppm in the diet for two years. Increased malignant spleen tumours in rats, no increase in tumours in mice.

Substance C

Rats and mice exposed orally to 6000–12 000 ppm in the diet for two years. Increased malignant liver tumours in both species.

Substance A is a reactive epoxide which is genotoxic *in vitro* and *in vivo*. On repeated inhalation exposure it produced inflammation of the respiratory tract. In the carcinogenicity studies conducted, long-term inhalation exposure produced inflammation and degeneration of the upper respiratory tract epithelium and malignant tumours in the upper respiratory tract. The interpretation reached is that the relative contributions to the carcinogenic process of genotoxicity and chronic epithelium inflammation are unclear, but both processes appear to be relevant to human health. Hence it is predicted that the carcinogenic hazard expressed in animals would also be expressed in humans under comparable (conceivable) circumstances. Resulting carcinogenicity classification: category 2.

Substance B is an aromatic amine which is genotoxic *in vitro* and at high doses has produced evidence of such activity *in vivo*. On repeated oral exposure in rats it produced damage to circulating red blood cells and effects in the spleen. In the carcinogenicity studies, long-term dietary exposure produced spleen damage and malignant tumours in rats. In similarly dosed mice these spleen effects did not occur and there were no significant increases in other tumours. The interpretation reached is that the spleen tumours in the rat may well have arisen as a result of chronic spleen damage. This did not occur in mice and it is not clear which is the best model for humans for this substance. Furthermore, it is questionable whether humans would continue to be chronically exposed to the substance once overt signs of red blood cell and spleen toxicity had appeared and hence whether the conditions ultimately resulting in the production of tumours in rats could conceivably by reproduced in humans. Hence uncertainty surrounds the relevance of the rat tumours for human health. Resulting carcinogenicity classification: category 3.

Substance C is a phthalate ester which is not directly genotoxic *in vitro* or *in vivo*. On repeated oral exposure it produces liver enlargement and proliferation of peroxisomes in liver cells. In the carcinogenicity studies conducted, long-term dietary exposure produced such liver changes and also malignant liver tumours. The interpretation reached is that the liver tumours arose as a result of the stimulation of peroxisome proliferation. It is known from other work that in comparison with rodent liver, the human liver is very much less responsive to this effect. Hence, as high dose levels were required to produce the carcinogenic effect in rodents, and as humans are predicted to be much less responsive, it is concluded that these rodent findings are not indicative of a realistic carcinogenic hazard for humans. Resulting carcinogenicity classification: not classified.

Another issue arising in toxicological hazard identification for existing substances is what to do when there are no data available on the substance itself in relation to a particular toxicological endpoint. Often one encounters substances on which there are no carcinogenicity or reproductive toxicity studies for instance, and for some substances the paucity of toxicological data available is severe, to the point of there being none at all!

In these cases, between the extremes of 'innocent until proven guilty' and 'suspect until proven clean' (it has been known for people to adopt these positions) there is surely a sensible compromise approach that can be taken to dealing with the toxicology of substances. This should involve consideration of:

- the chemical structure, physical form and physicochemical properties for toxicity clues (e.g. strong acids will burn, electrophilically reactive substances might well interact with DNA, very insoluble solids generally have low biological activity, large particles will not reach the deep lung);
- the known toxicological picture of analogues (although obviously one has to be careful in choosing the most appropriate analogues);
- the degree to which knowledge of some toxicological properties for a substance helps in predicting other toxicological properties (e.g. skin irritancy may be indicative of the potential for eye and upper respiratory tract irritancy; mutagenicity and repeated dose toxicity data, of both 'positive' and 'negative' types, may be helpful in predicting the carcinogenic potential).

A few examples of situations where it is suggested that certain aspects of hazard identification can be addressed, based on such predictions, are given below.

PREDICTION OF TOXICOLOGICAL HAZARD AND CONSEQUENT
EU CLASSIFICATION

Substance X is a liquid with the potential in use to become airborne, as liquid droplets and/or as a vapour. In relation to acute toxicity it has an oral LD50 (rats) of 100 mg/kg and a dermal LD50 (rats) of 700 mg/kg. It is therefore classified at Toxic (R25) on the basis of acute oral toxicity and Harmful (R21) on the basis of acute dermal toxicity. There are no acute inhalation toxicity data. Should (and if so, how should) the substance be classified in relation to acute inhalation toxicity on the basis that it could be predicted also to have 'classifiable' toxicity via this route? (Suggestion: Toxic (R23).)

Substance Y is chemically reactive towards biological molecules. As a consequence it is a direct-acting mutagen in vitro and in vivo. Another reflection of this reactivity is that it is strongly irritating towards biological tissue, provoking inflammation at sites of initial contact. Numerous other substances with these properties have been shown to be carcinogenic towards the respiratory tract in long-term inhalation exposure situations in experimental animals; for some such substances there is also direct evidence of respiratory tract cancer in humans. Substance Y has not been investigated for carcinogenicity. Should (and if so, how should) substance Y be classified for carcinogenic hazard on the basis of predictions made from other substances with analogous properties? (Suggestion: Category 3 (R40).)

Substance M is a dialkyl ether which undergoes relatively little metabolism. It is not mutagenic and on repeated exposure to high doses no significant tissue damage or tissue stimulation was seen. No carcinogenicity studies are available. How should classification with respect to carcinogenicity be assessed? (Suggestion: no indication of properties which would represent an underlying mechanism for carcinogenicity; conclude that the substance does not pose a carcinogenicity hazard.)

Substance N is an aliphatic ketone. No data are available concerning skin sensitization. However, it and its identified metabolites appear unreactive towards biological molecules. Data are available indicating a negative response for a structurally related ketone in a standard skin sensitization assay. How should classification with respect to skin sensitization be assessed? (Suggestion: no indication of the potential to form protein conjugates and negative data for an analogue; conclude that the substance does not pose a skin sensitization hazard.)

RISK ASSESSMENT

SUPPLY-SIDE PROGRAMMES

In recent years there has been an emergence of regulatory programmes requiring suppliers of chemical substances to go beyond hazard identification (classification and labelling) and to make an assessment of the risk posed to health once the substance is put onto the market. As with classification and labelling these programmes are not specifically focused on the workplace, but clearly the scenario of humans exposed at work is an important issue in the overall 'holistic' risk assessment demanded by the schemes.

For new substances, the EU 7th Amendment introduced the requirement for risk assessment of the chemicals notified to regulatory authorities; from a toxicology perspective this feature is probably the most significant change introduced into the EU new substances scene in moving from the era of the 6th Amendment (implemented in the UK by the Notification of New Substances Regulations 1982) (EEC, 1979; NONS, 1982) to that of the 7th Amendment (implemented in the UK by the Notification of New Substances Regulations 1993) (EEC, 1992; NONS, 1993). The specifications for such a risk assessment are given in the accompanying Risk Assessment Directive (EEC, 1993b) and an associated package of detailed technical guidance documents has also been produced.

In order to form a view on the risk to health in a particular situation one needs an idea of the level(s) of exposure involved. For new substances, when they are first notified at the pre-marketing stage, there is the obvious problem that there is no experience in use, either of the levels of exposure arising or of the impact on the exposed human population(s). Hence it is almost inevitable that for new substances, at least when they are first notified, exposure will have to be predicted/modelled on the basis of analogy and generic approaches. This situation and the relatively restricted package of toxicological data available initially, together with the other limitations on supply-side risk assessments (see below), have clear implications for the accuracy of any risk assessment for particular groups of exposed workers at individual sites. Workplace risk assessments are just beginning to be produced under this programme and, as yet, insufficient experience has been gained to examine properly how things are working out.

For existing substances, the OECD High Production Volume (HPV) chemicals programme has now been running for several years. The toxicology element of this programme is based on the principles of identifying the hazardous toxicological properties and assessing the risks to human health arising, for substances in the world market at high tonnage and for which it was believed that few data were available. The manner in which individual substances are covered by the programme entails a general sequence of:

- collection of available data, including toxicological and exposure data;
- identification of essential further information required in order to clarify the picture of the potential health, safety and environmental impact of the substance;
- gathering this further information, possibly entailing the commissioning of additional toxicity testing;
- detailing the hazardous properties of the substance, its dose-response characteristics, exposure data and the degree of risk involved for various sections of the human population (and the environment) encountering the substance.

The Existing Substances Regulation (ESR) (EEC, 1993a) is designed to deal with priority existing substances in Europe in a similar manner to the OECD HPV scheme. ESR also has an accompanying Risk Assessment Regulation and associated technical guidance documents. These are intended to specify in some detail the approach to be followed by regulatory authorities and industry in fulfilling the requirements of this programme. Again no experience has yet been gained of performing workplace risk assessments under ESR.

These existing substances schemes are founded on the notion that not enough is known about the hazardous properties and risks to health posed by chemicals that have been around for some time in the working environment and elsewhere. The associated guidance material for ESR specifies when and how further information on the hazardous properties should be sought, including the timing and structuring of new toxicological testing. It also deals with the provision, assessment and prediction of exposure data and the fusion of information on hazard and exposure in order to assess the risk to health posed by the substance.

The supply-side programmes are focused on manufacturers and suppliers of substances and reflect the philosophies of stewardship, cradle-to-grave and holistic management of chemicals. Each programme offers the regulators, as one potential outcome, the option of developing control measures to reduce the risk envisaged in any of the human exposure scenarios, including the workplace. However, from an occupational health standpoint, one difficulty that will undoubtedly arise is that of identifying and characterizing from the supply point all the potential workplaces, working practices and associated exposure situations that could arise with a particular substance. More difficult still will be the gathering of exposure data, an essential prerequisite to risk assessment, for all these situations. It is inevitable that the assessment of risk to health under these programmes cannot hope to embrace the detailed situation-specific features of a risk assessment related to local conditions performed by a chemical user under a programme such as the UK Control of Substances Hazardous to Health Regulations (COSHH, 1988).

Another issue arising from these supply-side schemes in relation to toxicity testing is the degree to which studies can be directed specifically towards addressing occupational health concerns, as opposed to other specific exposure scenarios or general approaches. For instance, where it is considered that repeated exposure toxicity data are lacking for a substance, necessitating further testing, should such testing employ the inhalation route if this appears to be the primary route of workplace exposure, or the oral route if there is interest in exposure via the environment, or both? Only experience with running these schemes in practice will indicate whether such issues represent a significant problem and, if so, how it may be resolved.

USER-SIDE PROGRAMMES

This heading is a convenient means of separating out this somewhat different facet of workplace risk assessment from the above discussion. However, the issues here also relate to risk assessments performed by chemical manufacturers in relation to their own workplaces and employees.

In the UK the COSHH Regulations require an employer to perform a risk assessment in relation to the circumstances prevailing at that particular workplace. Detailed knowledge of the specific conditions of each working environment under examination should improve considerably the reliability of the exposure assessment, and hence the risk assessment compared with a more generic supply-side assessment.

As the exercise is usually perceived from a toxicology standpoint, information on the hazardous properties of the substance in question will have been made available to the user via classification and labelling and safety data sheets. The user should then integrate this information with exposure considerations informing a view on the degree of risk involved in the specific situation and the appropriate measures to employ in limiting that risk.

From our experience as regulatory toxicologists, it has to be said that a significant proportion of safety data sheets are disappointing in the extent and quality of toxicological information offered. Some safety data sheets do not exhibit anything like the scope and depth of consideration which is necessary to give a reasonable picture of the toxicological properties of the substance. This must have knock-on consequences for the quality and reliability of the risk assessment performed by recipients of such information.

Much of the regulatory toxicology activity under COSHH (and other programmes based on similar concepts) has been directed towards establishment of occupational exposure limits for airborne substances, the framework for which is based on the principle of attempting to identify where possible exposure conditions entailing a very low/ insignificant risk of ill health. This area is discussed in more detail in the following section.

OCCUPATIONAL EXPOSURE LIMITS

The generation of lists of numerical airborne exposure levels, each proposed to represent an appropriate degree of control of occupational exposure to a chemical substance, has a long history stretching back to the early years of this century (Paull, 1984). Since the mid-1940s the Threshold Limit Values (TLVs) published by the American Conference of Government Industrial Hygienists (ACGIH, 1991) have been very influential all around the world in determining national positions on occupational exposure limits (OELs). Later, several European countries (Germany, the UK, The Netherlands, Denmark and Sweden) established their own systems for assessing chemicals for the purpose of deriving OELs. In recent years the EU, via its Directorate General V, has been seeking to develop a system for producing EU-wide OELs, building on the experiences and practices of the individual member states.

GENERAL FEATURES OF ESTABLISHING OELS

Setting meaningful and useful OELs is not solely a toxicological exercise. Rather, it is a multidisciplinary activity in which toxicology and toxicologists play one of the important roles. The following elements are required:

- an assessment of the toxicological picture;
- an assessment of the prevailing occupational hygiene situation and available practical options for control;
- a reliable and practical analytical technique;
- a policy framework within which the OEL is to sit.

The overall intention is obviously health protection. However, it is essential that in any OEL system there are precise criteria describing the degree of health protection which the OEL is intended to confer. It is unrealistic to expect that meaningful OELs offer cast-iron guarantees of absolute freedom from any biological effect for all possible members of the working population – the extent and quality of the toxicological information, the many uncertainties involved in the risk assessment process and the unachievability of extremely low exposures in many situations render impossible such a stringent standard of safety. A degree of protection something short of this, but nevertheless entailing at the very least avoidance of any significant risk of noteworthy health consequences, is the usual stated aim. Even then there may be some substances and situations where this cannot be achieved with confidence and it is important that any OEL system can pick up such cases and accommodate them in the form of a different type of OEL with different associated criteria. The UK two-category framework of Occupational Exposure Standards (OESs) and Maximum Exposure Limits (MELs) is an example of one such system. The OES is associated with a specific degree of health protection at that exposure level (HSE, 1993b); the MEL covers situations where such a degree of health protection is not assured at that exposure level.

TOXICOLOGY ELEMENT

The requirements of a toxicological assessment for the purposes of OEL setting are as follows. The known hazardous properties and dose-response characteristics for the substance are described. Data gaps are filled by prediction or, if this cannot be done with any confidence, knowledge gaps should be clearly identified to emphasize where areas of uncertainty lie. The aim is then to seek to identify a level of exposure which is considered to offer a level of health protection commensurate with criteria established for the OEL in question.

The nature of the principal toxicological effect(s) produced by the substance may necessitate specified controls for either the longer term aggregated dose (e.g. time-weighted average exposure over several hours) or short-term exposure of only a few minutes duration, or both. An attritional effect such as liver necrosis or lung fibrosis may be adequately controlled by the former type of limit, whereas an immediate effect such as sensory irritation, more dependent on airborne concentration than duration of exposure, requires tight control of short-term exposure. These factors need to be accommodated within an OEL system.

As a general principle, the toxicologist is usually faced with attempting to identify a No Observed Adverse Effect Level (NOAEL) from the data available in animals and/or humans. A 'health-assuring' OEL is then set somewhere at or below the NOAEL. The distance between the NOAEL and this type of OEL is variously described as an uncertainty factor, safety factor, safety margin, extrapolation factor, etc. Its purpose is to allow for the numerous uncertainties and inadequacies in our knowledge base at the time of the risk assessment. The issues involved in establishing an appropriate uncertainty factor are discussed later.

Frequently the toxicology task is rendered appreciably more difficult than it might appear from the above description. A paucity of data, poor quality information, conflicting data, absence of an identified NOAEL and the underlying general problems inherent in the three extrapolations (animal to human, route-to-route, high dose to low dose) usually confronting toxicologists all pose difficulties in this process. There is call for much professional judgement and, as a consequence, ample scope for dispute in assessment and interpretation. This renders absolutely essential the general principles of regulatory toxicology work discussed earlier in the chapter. The toxicological assessment must be available, clearly laid out and based on hard evidence and sound argument.

In some cases the toxicological picture, including the knowledge gaps, defeats the aim of identifying with confidence a level of exposure which is both sufficiently 'safe' and achievable in practice. This is often the situation in dealing with potent DNA-damaging (genotoxic/ mutagenic) chemicals with known or suspected consequential carcinogenic potential, examples being bis (chloromethyl) ether, ethylene oxide or o-toluidine. Respiratory sensitizers are another class of substance where such problems arise. The difficulty here is that there is currently no acceptable and widely used experimental test system for exploring this endpoint and therefore one is reliant almost exclusively on human clinical/medical information. In most cases this type of information does not permit the determination of dose – response characteristics for induction of a sensitized state and for triggering a response in hypersensitive individuals. Hence the need for an OEL system that can accommodate an inability to specify a 'believed to be safe' type of limit for all substances.

UNCERTAINTY FACTORS

In establishing an occupational exposure limit for which some assurance of freedom from health effects is given, one would wish to have:

(a) reliable data from human populations exposed to known levels of the substance, with at least one exposure level being a clear no-effect level for those health aspects that can be monitored; and

(b) confidence from toxicological information that other possible health effects that are difficult to detect in humans (e.g. mutagenicity, reproductive toxicity) give no cause for concern for the substance in question.

Unfortunately, almost invariably the toxicological information available on the substance is not sufficient in extent or quality to allow the direct and confident extraction of such a standard from the dataset. As stated above, the general approach used is to seek to identify a datapoint (usually the NOAEL) and to then apply an 'uncertainty factor' to allow for the uncertainties in moving to a lower level of exposure considered to meet the health protection criteria attached to the particular occupational exposure limit in question.

There are many issues which influence the size of the uncertainty factor. The principle issues are outlined below.

Extent and quality of toxicological information

In general the greater the amount of the data the lower would be the uncertainty. However this is by no means always the case, as sometimes a lot of information, some of which is conflicting, can produce a cloudy overall picture of the toxicology. Direct observations on humans will reduce the uncertainty, but if no firm data on human responsiveness are available, then there will always be some uncertainty concerning the relative sensitivity of humans compared with the animal species for which data are available. It is desirable that in setting an occupational exposure limit the toxicological data available relate to the inhalation route of exposure. As discussed above, if the only data available are for other routes of exposure, the uncertainty is increased and in some circumstances route-to-route extrapolation may be impossible. Better quality data give more confidence and hence less uncertainty than poorer quality data; the term 'quality' embraces the scope, rigorousness and conformity with accepted standards of the studies conducted, and the thoroughness of reporting of the findings. Finally, a preferred starting point for the derivation of an occupational exposure limit is a NOAEL. However, for some substances the data may demonstrate only a lowest observed adverse effect level (LOAEL), i.e. some adverse effects even at the lowest exposure level investigated. A larger uncertainty factor is likely to be required in this case.

Nature and severity of principal adverse effects

In general, the more severe the threat to life and well-being presented by the substance, the greater is the need to be confident in the health reassurance attached to the occupational exposure limit, and this will normally mean that a larger uncertainty factor is used. Other factors also have an influence, such as the slope of the dose – response curve and the degree of or lack of information on interspecies variation. A small uncertainty factor will apply where the principal effect of an airborne substance is mild sensory irritation which is rapidly and clearly apparent and readily and completely reversible on removal from exposure, particularly where there are reliable data for this endpoint. Relatively little interspecies variation would be expected for this local surface effect. In contrast, a much larger uncertainty factor is required where the principal effect of an airborne substance is severe developmental toxicity (e.g. birth defects) and where data for this endpoint are limited. This is a complex systemic effect with considerable scope for interspecies variability in toxicokinetics and toxicodynamics.

Nature of exposed population and exposure situation

In general the greater the variation in age, sex and underlying health condition of the exposed population, the greater will be the uncertainty factor required, to accommodate the considerable spread in responsiveness envisaged within the population. Another issue is the degree to which the particular exposure scenario is being kept in check. A smaller uncertainty factor is justifiable where there is assurance that exposure to the substance is actually being monitored and controlled to particular levels, where the health of the exposed population can be and is being monitored and where the ability to attribute any emerging health effect to a particular substance and to take effective remedial action is available. These features provide some justification for accepting smaller uncertainty factors in setting workplace 'health-based' exposure limits than, for instance, in setting environmental standards for the general population as a whole.

Degree of control achievable

There is not just one possible level of exposure that can be argued as meeting the health protection criteria associated with the occupational exposure limit in question. Rather, there are many candidates for 'appropriate' exposure levels, going back from the starting data-point (e.g. NOAEL) towards zero exposure. It is undoubtedly true that the size of the uncertainty factor, i.e. how low an occupational exposure limit is set, is influenced by the type of control options available, the extent of control achievable in the particular exposed population and the associated sociological and economic impact of the controls envisaged. Where a large uncertainty factor can be used to give absolute certainty of safety, or where a large uncertainty factor would effectively result in a ban or very severe restriction on the use of the substance, with relatively minor repercussions, then large uncertainty factors can be applied liberally (e.g. with a new fragrance or a colourant for foodstuffs). For the vast majority of industrial situations such freedom does not exist and for practical, technical and socioeconomic reasons the size of uncertainty factors must be lower, whilst still maintaining the aim of eliminating or minimizing the risk to health.

Clearly many issues must be taken into account in determining an uncertainty factor. Some, but not all, are scientific issues and even for these there is often not a scientific data-based solution readily available, due to lack of information. The general toxicological literature abounds with statements that it is conventional in regulatory work to use uncertainty factors based on specified contributions from individual elements, e.g. a factor of 10 to allow for interspecies variation, another factor of 10 to allow for intraspecies variation, etc. and that these individual elements are multiplicative. Such schemes have been proposed mainly for non-occupational exposure situations (Lu, 1988: Rubery, Barlow and Steadman, 1990; Renwick, 1993). However, in reality in the occupational context there are severe problems with such an approach, both in terms of a lack of scientific basis for the factors used and the impracticality of the very large uncertainty factors so generated when one applies the approach to the relatively weak toxicological databases available on many substances. In practice uncertainty factors for occupational exposure limits setting have evolved by committee 'expert judgement' and precedent. An example of the derivation of an OES, with its associated uncertainty factor, for cyclohexane, debated within the UK system during 1990, is given below.

EXAMPLE OF AN OCCUPATIONAL EXPOSURE STANDARD
DERIVED WITHIN THE UK SYSTEM FOR ESTABLISHING
OCCUPATIONAL EXPOSURE LIMITS

Cyclohexane; 100 ppm (8h TWA) OES
There is a reasonable amount of toxicological data available in animals, approximating to the base-set available on initial notification of a 'new substance'; negligible human data were available.

In relation to the areas of sensitization and mutagenicity/carcinogenicity, where positive findings give rise to most difficulties in establishing 'safe' levels of exposure, there are no actual experimental data on sensitization potential. However, the non-electrophilic nature of cyclohexane and its identified metabolites and the absence of any reports of sensitization in humans in situations where repeated skin and inhalation exposure must have occurred suggest that cyclohexane is not a sensitizer. A package of mutagenicity tests indicates that cyclohexane is not mutagenic and there is no reason to suspect any significant carcinogenic activity. There is no information on its potential to produce reproductive effects.

Only one general repeated exposure study is available, involving rabbits exposed by inhalation to 434, 787, or 3335 ppm cyclohexane for 6 hours per day, 5 days per week for 10 weeks or 437 ppm, 8 hours per day, 5 days per week for up to 26 weeks. The investigation incorporated clinical examination, haematology and histopathology. However, the work is quite old (1943) and its conduct and reporting clearly do not reach the standards of a contemporary 28/90-day study. A NOAEL of 434 ppm was evident.

This study was crucial to the establishment of an OES of 100 ppm (8h TWA). This 8h TWA value is about four times lower than the 434 ppm NOAEL, and eight times lower than a LOAEL of 787 ppm, which produced ill-characterized, slight histopathology changes in the liver and kidney.

An analysis has recently been produced of the uncertainty factors involved in the establishment of OES values for substances considered within the UK OELs system during the period 1990–93 (Fairhurst, 1995). It is an unfortunate fact that for the vast majority of substances there is a paucity of well-documented health experience associated with the use of occupational exposure limits within the workplace. Until such information becomes available it is difficult to assess scientific 'correctness' of the uncertainty factors used, in respect of their absolute numerical values. Indeed, given the number of people exposed to chemicals at work, the range of substances involved and the considerable period of time over which such exposures have been occurring, the paucity of well-documented information on human experience at known levels of chemical exposure is disappointing. Ultimately, such experience is vital to an accurate appreciation of the toxicology situation in any workplace.

REFERENCES

ACGHH (1991) *Documentation of the Threshold Limit Values and Biological Exposure Indices*, 6th edn, vols 1–3, American Conference of Governmental Hygienists Inc., Circinnati, OH, USA.

CHIP (1993) The Chemicals (Hazard Information and Packaging) Regulations 1993 (Statutory Instruments 1993, No. 1746), HMSO, London, UK.

COSHH (1988) The Control of Substances Hazardous to Health Regulations 1988 (Statutory Instruments 1988, No. 1657), HMSO, London, UK.

ECETOC (1987) Technical Report No. 26: The Assessment of Carcinogenic Hazard for Human Beings Exposed to Methylene Chloride. European Chemical Industry Ecology and Toxicology Centre, Brussels, Belgium.

EEC (1967) Council Directive 67/548/EEC on the Approximation of the Laws, Regulations and Administrative Provisions Relating to the Classification, Packaging and Labelling of Dangerous Substances.

EEC (1979) Council Directive 79/831/EEC, Amending for the Sixth Time Directive 67/548/EEC on the Approximation of the Laws, Regulations and Administrative Provisions Relating to the Classification, Packaging and Labelling of Dangerous Substances.

EEC (1988) Council Directive 88/379/EEC on the Approximation of the Laws, Regulations and Administrative Provisions of the Member States relating to the Classification, Packaging and Labelling of Dangerous Preparations.

EEC (1992) Council Directive 92/32/EEC, Amending for the Seventh Time Directive 67/548/EEC on the Approximation of the Laws, Regulations and Administrative Provisions Relating to the Classification, Packaging and Labelling of Dangerous Substances.

EEC (1993a) Council Regulation (EEC) No. 793/93 of 23 March 1993 on the Evaluation and Control of the Risks of Existing Substances.

EEC (1993b) Commission Directive 93/67/EEC, Laying Down the Principles for Assessment of Risks to Man and the Environment of Substances Notified in Accordance with Council Directive 67/548/EEC.

Elkins, H.B. (1959) *The Chemistry of Industrial Toxicology*, 2nd edn, John Wiley and Sons, New York.

Fairhurst, S. (1995) Application of uncertainty factors in deriving UK occupational exposure standards. *The Annals of Occupational Hygiene* (in press).

HSC (1993) Approved Supply List: Information Approved for the Classification and Labelling of Substances and Preparations Dangerous for Supply: Chemicals (Hazard Information and Packaging) Regulations 1993. HMSO, London.

HSE (1993a) EH64: Occupational Exposure Limits: Criteria Document Summaries, HMSO, London.

HSE (1993b) EH40/93: Occupational Exposure Limits 1993, HMSO, London.

Lu, F.C. (1988) Acceptable daily intake: inception, evolution and application. *Regulatory and Applied Toxicology*, **8**, 45–60.

NONS (1982) The Notification of New Substances Regulations 1982 (Statutory Instruments 1982, No. 1496), HMSO, London.

NONS (1993) The Notification of New Substances Regulations 1993 (Statutory Instruments 1993, No. 3050), HMSO, London.

Patty, F.A. (ed.) (1963) *Industrial Hygiene and Toxicology*, 2nd revised edn, **11**, Interscience Publishers, New York.

Paull, J.M. (1984) The origin and basis of threshold limit values. *American Journal of Industrial Medicine*, **5**, 227–38.

Renwick, A.G. (1993) Data-derived safety factors for the evaluation of food additives and environmental contaminants. *Food Additives and Contaminants*, **10**, 275–306.

Rubery, E.D., Barlow, S.M., Steadman, J.H. (1990) Criteria for setting quantitative estimates of acceptable intake of chemicals in food in the UK. *Food Additives and Contaminants*, **7**, 287–302.

Sax, N.I. and Levis, R.J. Snr (eds) (1989) *Dangerous Properties of Industrial Materials*, 7th edn, vols 1–3, Van Nostrand Reinhold, New York.

Ergonomics in the workplace

7

Ted Megaw

DEFINITION AND SCOPE OF ERGONOMICS

There are numerous definitions of ergonomics and the following one, which is a slightly modified version of the one provided by Murrell (1965), captures the essence of a majority of them:

> Ergonomics can be defined as the scientific study of the relationship between people and their working environments. In this sense, the term environment is taken to cover not only the ambient environment in which they work but also their tools and materials, their methods of work and the organization of their work, either as an individual or within a working group. All these are related to the nature of the people themselves: to their abilities, capacities and limitations.

There are several interdependent aims of ergonomics, the most significant of which are to:

- reduce health and safety risks;
- ensure appropriate workloads, both physical and mental, so that on the one hand jobs are not boring and monotonous, and on the other hand they are not overdemanding;
- develop 'usable' systems and products;
- achieve a good quality of working life and job satisfaction;
- increase productivity, not just by reducing direct costs, for example, by increasing output rates, but also by decreasing absenteeism and turnover, and improving quality.

While these aims may appear to be mainly concerned with manufacturing and commercial environments, it should be emphasized that ergonomics is equally applicable to the service industries including education, to the home including domestic activities and homeworking, to sports and leisure activities, to transportation systems, to military and space environments, as well as to agriculture which involves over half the world's working population. Central to ergonomics is the belief that account should be taken of the vast differences between the physical and mental capabilities of people. Traditionally, especially in manufacturing environments, there has been a marked tendency for jobs to be designed only for physically fit young or middle-aged males. However, less than a half of the working population in the UK falls into this category as a result of an increase in the employment of women, albeit often on a part-time basis, and of a general ageing of the population as well as the legal requirements to employ disabled people.

In some circles, particularly in the USA, the terms 'human factors' or 'human factors engineering' have been preferred. Although there have been some claims that there are subtle differences in the definitions of human factors and ergonomics, it is generally now accepted that the terms can be freely interchanged. The first professional society, the Ergonomics Research Society, was set up in the UK in 1949. In 1976 the title was changed to the Ergonomics Society in order to emphasize the practical nature of the subject. The largest national society is currently the Human Factors and Ergonomics Society (formerly the Human Factors Society) which was established in North America in 1955. There are now over 30 individual national societies encompassing over 15 000 individual members and these societies are brought together under the auspices of the International Ergonomics Association.

What is clear from the definition given at the beginning of this chapter is that the scope of ergonomics is enormous, and this can be appreciated by taking a simple systems view of the subject as shown in Figure 7.1. Interface design incorporates much of what is often referred to as knobs-and-dials ergonomics, but more recently has been extended by the developments in computer interfaces. Typical interface design includes a consideration of the following topics:

- display and control design
- display and control layout
- warning and alarm systems
- information presentation
- system feedback and adaptation
- furniture and equipment design
- general workplace design.

In order to perform their tasks, operators frequently require assistance from a number of support resources. These include:

- manuals, instructions and help documentation

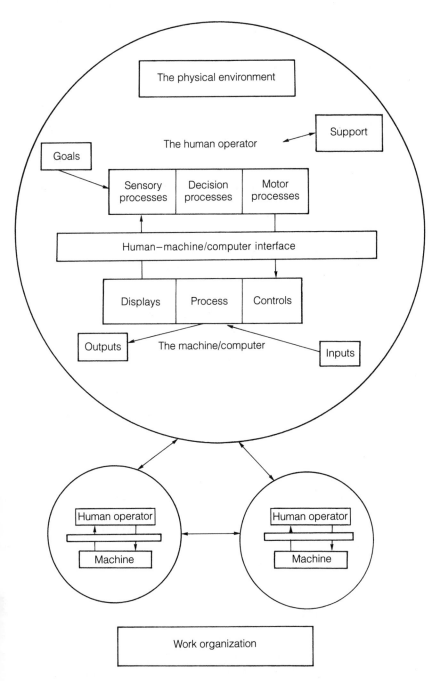

Figure 7.1 The various components of the study of ergonomics.

- work procedures, especially for fault diagnosis and maintenance activities
- human support
- decision support systems including expert systems
- training.

Naturally, the human–machine/computer interface does not reside within a vacuum. There is a need to consider the physical environment as any deviation from optimal conditions is likely to degrade operator performance. The most obvious environmental factors concern lighting, noise, vibration and climate but under very special conditions factors such as acceleration forces, barometric pressure and gaseous mixtures need to be considered. Ideally the ergonomist attempts to control the physical environment so that conditions are kept optimal or as near optimal as possible. In those cases where this is impossible, ergonomics becomes concerned with the design of protective clothing and equipment. However, it should be emphasized that the use of protective clothing and equipment often leads to a decrease in human performance and can create additional problems of safety, and consequently should only be adopted when there is no obvious means of improving the quality of the physical environment. In addition, the physical environment is taken to include the design of the physical space requirements as well as facilities layout.

Finally there is the need to consider those factors concerned with the broader aspects of the job. These include factors such as:

- the allocation of tasks and jobs between people and the machine or computer systems
- duration of work and rest periods
- the organization of shift work
- the organization of team or group work
- job design involving job enlargement, job satisfaction and job characteristics
- the design of communication and information systems, particularly for distributed work
- payment systems
- the implementation of technological change.

INFLUENCES IN THE DEVELOPMENT OF ERGONOMICS

It is generally accepted that the major development of ergonomics arose out of problems which came to light during the Second World War, problems such as the design of controls for anti-aircraft guns, the space requirements for fighter aircraft pilots, and the duration of work periods for radar operators. However, there were some notable examples of the application of ergonomics before the term ergonomics was established. For example, one can see the origins of industrial ergonomics in the work of the Industrial Fatigue Research Board in the UK in the 1920s. Despite these various influences the impact of ergonomics remained comparatively ineffective outside the military context for a long time. Within service and manufacturing industries this was partly a consequence of the trade unions not taking ergonomics on board, often preferring to accept dirt pay for working in hazardous environments, and partly a consequence of management not appreciating the cost-benefits of applying ergonomics and often dismissing ergonomics on the grounds that it is only concerned with problems of seating and the like.

However, on 29th March 1979, an incident occurred at the Three Mile Island (TMI) Unit 2 nuclear plant near Harrisburg, Pennsylvania which was to have a marked influence on the development of ergonomics. Although the outcome of the incident was not as horrific (no loss of life resulted from the incident) as many of the more recent disasters such as Bhopal (where at least 3500 people were killed and more than 200 000 inhabitants were injured), Chernobyl, Zeebrugge, Kegworth and King's Cross, the implications were to be far reaching. For the first time a whole range of ergonomics related system features were publicly implicated as leading to the human error which finally led to a partial core meltdown in the PWR reactor. These features included poor information presentation and control room design, confusing alarm systems, incorrect maintenance, inadequate training, confusing operator procedures, problems over shift work, diffusion of responsibility, and mismanagement. For a fuller analysis of the TMI incident readers are referred to Perrow (1984), Rubinstein and Mason (1979) and Megaw (1991). While it is self-evident that highlighting the causes of the incident did not prevent the occurrence of subsequent disasters, there is little doubt that the resulting increased awareness of the importance of ergonomics has reduced the risks associated with the proliferation of high-risk technologies.

In addition to TMI, some other important influences should be noted. One of these centres on the dramatic rise in the use of computer-based products. This is an area where ergonomics has played a crucial role in the design and evaluation of usable products to the extent that the claim that a product has incorporated ergonomics into the design process is frequently used as a major marketing point. The same development can be seen with telecommunications products. Another major influence has been associated with the increase in reports of musculoskeletal disorders accompanying several forms of repetitive physical work and static postures. Most significant of these disorders are those to the back arising from the adoption of poor manual lifting and handling procedures as well as working in awkward postures. Although not due solely to a disregard of ergonomics factors, it is worth emphasizing that 46.5 million working days were lost from back pain in 1989 at an estimated cost of £2000 million (Stubbs and Buckle, 1991). The more celebrated musculo-skeletal disorders are those now commonly referred to as repetitive strain injuries (RSI) or more correctly as cumulative trauma disorders (Putz-Anderson, 1988). Compensation claims for RSI in Australia, including cases arising from computer keyboard work, amounted to A$400 million by 1985. While compensation claims for RSI have declined in Australia over recent years they are set to accelerate in the UK as a result of the successful compensation claim of £79 000 achieved by a typist for the Inland Revenue early in 1993.

LEGISLATION

Because of the apparent lack of commitment to ergonomics exhibited by both management and unions in the UK, legislation can be seen as an important means by which to encourage a more serious consideration of ergonomic factors in the workplace. Although the Health and Safety at Work etc. Act (1974) went some way to increasing awareness of the responsibility of management and workers to health and safety issues, the impact regarding the introduction of ergonomics was minimal. However, recent legislation, much of it arising out of European directives, is much more explicit in demanding the application of ergonomics and it is likely to be of significance to a majority of workers in both manufacturing and commercial organizations. The HSE regulations which directly implement EC directives are:

- Provision and Use of Work Equipment Regulations 1992, implementing EC Directive 89/655/EEC;
- Health and Safety (Display Screen Equipment) Regulations 1992, implementing EC Directive 90/270/EEC;
- Manual Handling Operations Regulations 1992, implementing EC Directive 90/269/EEC;
- Personal Protective Equipment at Work Regulations 1992, implementing EC Directive 89/686/EEC.

At the same time, although not implementing an EC directive, the HSE published the Workplace (Health, Safety and Welfare) Regulations 1992.

These came into force on 1st January 1993, along with the Management of Health and Safety at Work Regulations 1992 which brings the above regulations into the general context of the Health and Safety at Work etc. Act 1974.

As an example of the scope of this new legislation, the Health and

Safety (Display Screen Equipment) Regulations 1992 will be described in some detail. It is estimated that at least 5 million workers will be affected by them. There are nine regulations which can be summarized as follows.

Regulation 1. Citation, commencement, interpretation and application

This regulation is concerned with defining terms and, in particular, establishing which display screen equipment is covered and who is a display screen user or operator. The regulation is slightly ambivalent concerning home working, although it definitely covers employees who are required to work at a workstation in their homes. In terms of usage, a user or operator can usually be considered as someone who works with display screen equipment for continuous periods in excess of an hour on a daily basis. Displays whose main use is to show television or film pictures are not included. It is probable that people who use TV screens for surveillance work and computer-supported cooperative work are covered.

Regulation 2. Analysis of workstations to assess and reduce risks

To a large extent, the need to assess and reduce risks is already implied in the Health and Safety at Work etc. Act 1974 as well as made explicit in the Management of Health and Safety at Work Regulations 1992. The risks normally considered in this context are those associated with upper limb musculo-skeletal problems, visual problems, and fatigue and stress. Other concerns include epilepsy, facial dermatitis, electro-magnetic radiation related problems and the effects on pregnant women.

Regulation 3. Requirements for workstations

This regulation lays down the conditions to be taken to ensure that workstations meet the requirements laid down in the Schedule to the Regulations. Workstations first put into service before 1st January 1993 must meet these requirements by 31st December 1996, while those introduced after 31st December 1992 must meet the requirements at the time they are put into service. However, it should be emphasized that even those workstations introduced before 1st January 1993 must comply with the other regulations and the Health and Safety at Work etc. Act 1974 so that a risk assessment must be performed as stated in regulation 2 and corrective action taken to ensure that the risks are reduced to the lowest extent reasonably practicable. The Schedule covers the human–computer interface including both hardware and software features. These include the characteristics of the screen, the keyboard, the workplace furniture, the information presentation and the system feedback. The Schedule also covers physical environmental factors such as lighting, noise, climate and the space requirements for the workstation. The Schedule does not cover work organization issues. It should be realized that all the requirements listed in the Schedule should not necessarily be met by all workstations. For example, many operators in control rooms monitor displays while standing, in which case there is no obligation to provide for that particular workstation a chair, a footrest, a work desk or a document holder.

Regulation 4. Daily work routine of users

This regulation mainly concerns the allocation of rest breaks. These should be taken before the onset of fatigue, should be included as a part of working time, should be frequent and of short duration rather than long and infrequent, and should be informal rather than formal. It is also recommended that individuals should be allowed discretion as to how they carry out their tasks and over their pace of work.

Regulation 5. Eyes and eyesight

According to this regulation, users can request an eye or eyesight test, as defined in the Opticians Act 1989, to be paid for by the employers. Employers are also liable to pay for the appropriate corrective appliances where normal corrective appliances are not suitable. In practice this means providing corrective appliances for intermediate work (i.e. for viewing distances of 50–60 cm).

Regulation 6. Provision of training

Employers are required to provide users with adequate health and safety training in the use of any workstation they may be required to work at and, if necessary, with retraining if any modifications are made to their workstation. This training is mainly concerned with the risks mentioned under regulation 2. An important point to make is that any risk assessment carried out according to regulation 2 should only be done after users have received the appropriate training.

Regulation 7. Provision of information

This reflects the requirement under the Management of Health and Safety at Work Regulations 1992 for employers to provide information on risks to safety and health to all their employees. This relates to the information covered under regulations 2 to 6.

Regulation 8. Exemption certificates

This applies to military employees.

Regulation 9. Extension outside the UK

This is covered by the Health and Safety at Work etc. Act 1974.

A further significant development within the statutory framework in the USA has been MANPRINT (Manpower and Personnel Integration). MANPRINT is a military system procurement initiative adopted by the US army. It integrates six areas of user concern – human factors engineering, manpower, personnel, training, health hazards, and system safety. The programme extends beyond military systems and can be applied to all products and systems including cars, aircraft, ships, control rooms, automated manufacturing, telecommunications, computers and medical equipment (Booher, 1990). Currently, the MANPRINT philosophy is being adopted by the MoD in the UK.

STANDARDS AND GUIDELINES

Typical of most legislation is the absence of objective criteria by which to evaluate whether or not the law is being adhered to. This lack of comprehensive criteria is reflected in the Offices, Shops and Railway Premises Act 1963 which provides some sporadic criteria on environmental conditions. For example, regarding space requirements, the Act stipulates a minimum of $3.7\,m^2$ per occupant. In respect of climate, the Act states that if work does not involve severe physical work, a temperature of at least 16°C must be achieved after the first hour of work. When it comes to lighting, the Act resorts to vague phrases such as 'Effective provision shall be made for securing and maintaining ... sufficient and suitable lighting, whether natural or artificial ... ' (pp. 6–7). Noise is covered by separate legislation which now provides comparatively detailed criteria – the Noise at Work Regulations 1989. According to these regulations employees can request personal ear protectors when their daily personal noise exposure is between 85 and 90 dB(A), and if the daily exposure is above 90 dB(A) employers must take steps to reduce the exposure levels so far as is reasonably practicable, otherwise than by the provision of personal ear protectors. If, as a result of taking such steps, the exposure values are still above 90 dB(A), employers must, by the provision of personal ear protectors, so far as is reasonably practicable, bring the exposure level to below 90 dB(A).

Because of this general lack of objective criteria contained within the legislation itself, it is necessary to make reference to various standards and guideline documents. For example, when considering the Health and Safety (Display Screen Equipment) Regulations 1992, there are many relevant publications, the most obvious being BS 7179 (1990) and ISO 9241 (1992). BS 7179 is divided into six parts:

Part 1. Introduction
Part 2. Recommendations for the design of office tasks
Part 3. Specification for visual displays
Part 4. Specification for keyboards
Part 5. Specification for VDT workstations
Part 6. Code of practice for the design of VDT work environments.

The information for Part 5 is derived from two other standards concerned with office workstations, BS 5940 (1980) and BS 3044 (1990). It is probable that BS 7179 will at some time be superseded by ISO 9241. ISO 9241 is considerably more detailed than BS 7179, and includes much of the material contained in the American National Standard for Human Factors Engineering of Visual Display Terminal Workstations (ANSI/HFS 100-1988). Many of the 17 parts to ISO 9241, listed below, are as yet only draft international standards and some are still in committee draft form:

Part 1. General introduction
Part 2. Guidance on task requirements
Part 3. Visual display requirements
Part 4. Keyboard requirements
Part 5. Workstation layout and postural requirements
Part 6. Environmental requirements
Part 7. Display requirements with reflections
Part 8. Requirements for displayed colours
Part 9. Requirements for non-keyboard input devices
Part 10. Dialogue principles
Part 11. Usability statements
Part 12. Presentation of information
Part 13. User guidance
Part 14. Menu dialogues
Part 15. Command dialogues
Part 16. Direct manipulation dialogues
Part 17. Form filling dialogues.

While space does not permit a full description of all the other standards and guidelines which have a direct bearing on ergonomics, the following list includes what are probably the most significant documents. Included with these are a number of relevant ergonomics textbooks.

General

ISO 6385, 1991; DEF Stan 00-25, 1984–1992; Adams, 1989; Oborne, 1987; Pheasant, 1991; Sanders and McCormick, 1992; Wilson and Corlett, 1990.

Equipment and workplace design

BS 4099, 1986; BS 4467, 1991; BS 5304, 1988; BS 5378, 1980; BS 7231, 1990; Astrand and Rodahl, 1986; Pheasant, 1986; Woodson, Tillman and Tillman, 1992.

The physical environment

CIBSE, 1978; CIBSE, 1994; BS 6841, 1987; BS 6482, 1987; Kryter, 1985; Parsons, 1993; Griffin, 1990.

Work organization

Davis and Taylor, 1979; Boddy and Buchanan, 1986; Eason, 1988; Monk and Folkard, 1992; Swezey and Salas, 1992; Salvendy and Karwowski, 1994.

AN APPLICATION OF ERGONOMICS IN THE WORKPLACE: WORK-RELATED MUSCULO-SKELETAL DISORDERS

Work-related musculo-skeletal disorders are often divided into three, though closely related, classes of problem:

- manual lifting and handling operations
- working postures
- cumulative trauma disorders.

MANUAL LIFTING AND HANDLING OPERATIONS

A good introduction to manual lifting and handling tasks is provided by Mital, Nicholson and Ayoub (1993). They cover not only repetitive lifting tasks but also tasks requiring pushing, pulling, carrying or simply holding. In terms of legislation within the UK, the most significant document is the Manual Handling Operations Regulations 1992. The essence of these regulations is to be found in regulation 4 – duties of employers. This regulation follows on from the application of the Management of Health and Safety at Work Regulations 1992 when a general assessment reveals a possible risk to employees from the manual handling of loads. Regulation 4 proposes a hierarchy of preventive measures. Initially, the need for employees to undertake manual handling operations which involve a risk of their being injured should be avoided either by totally eliminating the load handling operations or, if that is not possible, by automating or mechanizing the operations. If it is not considered reasonably practicable to avoid the need, then a risk assessment should be undertaken taking account of the factors specified in Schedule 1 to the Regulations. The questions that must be considered according to the Schedule relate to the task, the loads, the working environment, the capabilities of the individuals, and finally any other significant factors (e.g. the need to wear protective clothing such as gloves). Having carried out a risk assessment, the final stage involves the requirement to take the appropriate steps to reduce the risk of injury to the lowest level reasonably practicable. This can be achieved by applying general ergonomics principles. In the HSE Guidance on the Regulations (HSE, 1992), there is a checklist (Appendix 2) to help with the risk assessment and reduction processes. What is absent from the Regulations and the accompanying guidance are recommendations regarding safe limits for lifting as a function of various task factors.

The most comprehensive guidelines for recommended weight limits (RWLs) for lifting tasks have been developed by the US National Institute for Occupational Safety and Health (NIOSH, 1981; 1991). The lifting equations of NIOSH relating RWL to a number of task parameters are based on three criteria derived from the application of biomechanics, work physiology and psychophysics. The three respective criteria are:

- a maximum disc compression force of 3.4 kN (350 kg)
- a maximum energy expenditure of 2.2–4.7 kcal min^{-2} (depending on the vertical location of the lift and the duration of continuous lifting)
- a maximum acceptable weight of 75% of all female workers and 99% of all male workers.

As a result of the application of these criteria, RWLs can be established for a variety of lifting tasks which can be performed by nearly all healthy workers over a working day without any increased risk of developing low back pain. According to the revised equation (NIOSH, 1991), RWLs (separate RWLs are calculated for the point of origin of the lift and the final destination of the lift) can be calculated by including a number of multiplying factors so that

$$RWL = LC \times HM \times VM \times DM \times AM \times FM \times CM$$

where

LC = load constant   = 23 kg
HM = horizontal multiplier = (25/H)

VM = vertical multiplier $= (1 - (0.003|V - 75|))$
DM = distance multiplier $= (0.82 + (4.5/D))$
AM = asymmetric multiplier = $(1 - (0.0032A))$
FM = frequency multiplier (a function of work duration, vertical location of the lift and lifts min^{-2})
CM = coupling multiplier (a function of the quality of handles and the vertical location of the lift)

and where

H = horizontal distance of hands from midpoint between the ankles, measured at the origin and the destination of the lift (cm)
V = vertical distance of the hands from the floor, measured at the origin and the destination of the lift (cm)
D = vertical travel distance between the origin and the destination of the lift (cm)
A = angle of asymmetry (angular displacement of the load from the sagittal plane measured at the origin and the destination of the lift (degrees).

For a fuller account of the development of the revised NIOSH guidelines, readers are referred to Waters *et al.* (1993). What should be emphasized is that the NIOSH equation is only really applicable to tasks where lifting is a major component of a person's job, and does not take account of the other handling operations found in many jobs.

POSTURE

Although the problems associated with posture are far more general than those associated with lifting tasks, for example they concern basic issues in workplace design, there is no legislation covering posture other than that contained within legislation requiring a general risk assessment. Fortunately a number of simple ergonomics tools have been developed, particularly by Scandinavian researchers, to identify risks associated with posture. These tools rely on simple observation techniques which can be applied with very little training. Typical of these is OWAS (the Ovako Working posture Analysis System), developed in Finland by Karhu, Kansi and Kuorinka (1977). The essential features of this system are shown in Figure 7.2(a) where both the posture set and a typical evaluation chart are illustrated. In practice, four levels of risk are identified as a function of a number of postural factors: back posture, upper-limb posture, lower-limb posture, and the degree of strength required. The four levels of risk relate to how soon after the assessment remedial action should be taken: no action necessary, action in the near future, action soon, action immediately.

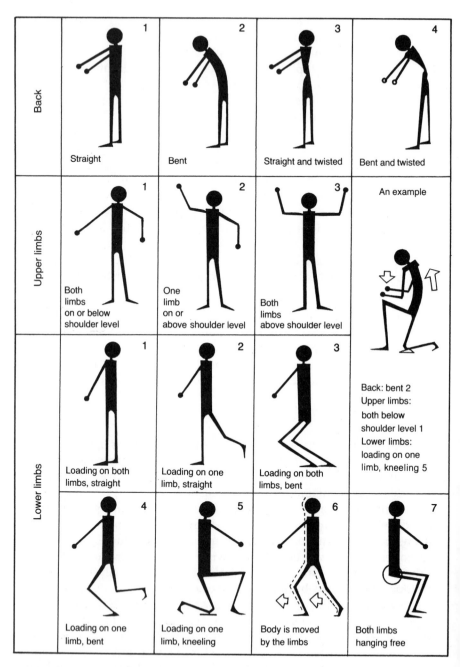

Figure 7.2 (a) The OWAS posture set, (b) A typical posture evaluation chart, Reproduced with permission from Wilson and Corlett (1990).

| Worker | | | Duration (min.) | | | | Number of observations | | | | | | | | | | | | | | | | |
| Research worker | | | Observation (min.)
Interval (min.) | | | | | | | | | | | | | | | | | | | | |

	Back	Upper extre-mities	Lower extremities – use of strength																				
			1			2			3			4			5			6			7		
			1	2	3	1	2	3	1	2	3	1	2	3	1	2	3	1	2	3	1	2	3
Total number of observations at work	1	1																					
		2																					
		3																					
	2	1																					
		2																					
		3																					
	3	1																					
		2																					
		3																					
	4	1																					
		2																					
		3																					
Not working	Pause						Waiting						No observation										

Not harmful – no action
Some strain – near future
Major strain – as soon as possible
Harmful – do at once

Figure 7.2 *Continued*

The method requires several observations to be made so that the percentage time associated with the various postures adopted during the work task can also be assessed. Examples of the application of OWAS include bricklaying (Kivi and Mattila, 1991), work in garages (Kant, Notermans and Borm, 1990) and nursing (Engels, Landeweerd and Kant, 1994).

In a more recent study by Hickson and Megaw (1994), both OWAS and the revised NIOSH lifting formula were used to investigate lifting and postural problems on a car assembly line. The task involved fitting the vehicle's steering rack assembly to the bulkhead and the steering column while the car was moving on a bogey just above floor level, a task acknowledged by both unions and management as being particularly hazardous. The OWAS analysis revealed that the problem was mainly due to the need to have the back in a bent and twisted posture with both arms often below the shoulder. Application of the NIOSH formula revealed that the RWLs for the steering rack assembly with the existing lifting method was about 4 kg for both the origin and the destination of the lift, a value considerably less than the actual weight of the steering rack assembly which was 11 kg. To improve the task, it was proposed that the fitting operation should be performed at some stage during the assembly when the cars were raised above the operators so that the work could be performed with the operators assuming a vertical posture by approaching the car from underneath rather than from the front. By simulating these proposed conditions a significant reduction in the risk of injury from bad posture was identified by the application of OWAS. The RWLs with the new method of presenting the cars to the operators were estimated as 11.6 kg at the origin and 10.1 kg at the destination of the lift, values close to the actual weight of the component.

Another useful tool for investigating problems of postural load is the Standardized Nordic Questionnaires (Kuorinka et al., 1987). In particular, these questionnaires provide a standard format for gathering information on musculo-skeletal problems so that comparisons could be made between different studies as well as facilitating long-term epidemiological analyses. A much shorter checklist for identifying risk factors due to awkward postures has been developed by Keyserling, Brouwer and Silverstein (1992). A survey method which has been designed more specifically for aiding the assessment requirements of the new UK legislation is described by McAtamney and Corlett (1993).

CUMULATIVE TRAUMA DISORDERS (CTDS)

These disorders are mainly characterized by the fact they are sustained through repeated actions, although the frequency with which a particular action must be performed to be considered repeated is open to debate. An operational definition of CTDs has been provided by Kroemer (1989):

> CTD is a collective term for syndromes characterized by discomfort, impairment, disability or persistent pain in joints, muscles, tendons and other soft tissues, with or without physical manifestations. It is caused by repetitive motions including vibrations, sustained or constrained postures, and forceful movements at work or leisure. (p. 274)

The terms over-use injury and repetitive strain injury are often used to describe the same conditions. CTDs usually occur to the hands and wrists, arms and elbows, shoulder and neck and occasionally leg and foot. They include tendon disorders such as tenosynovitis, nerve disorders such as carpal tunnel syndrome, vascular disorders such as white finger, and neurovascular disorders such as thoracic outlet syndrome. Although repetitive loading may cause problems to the back, it is usual in the literature to distinguish problems arising from manual materials lifting and handling when discussing CTDs. An extensive list of the various CTDs and their associated occupations and job characteristics has been collated by Putz-Anderson (1988) and a modified version of that list prepared by Kroemer (1989) is shown in Table 7.1.

As is the case when investigating postural problems at work, there is no specific legislation concerned with CTDs other than general legislation associated with risk assessment and compensation claims. On the other hand, there is general agreement on the ergonomics measures that should be taken to avoid CTDs (Kroemer, 1989). These are:

- avoid job activities with many repetitions, e.g. where the cycle time is less than 30 sec;
- avoid work that requires prolonged or repetitive exertion of more than 30% of the operator's muscle strength available for that activity;
- avoid body segments adopting extreme postures, e.g. severe beñing of the wrist;
- avoid work that forces workers to maintain the same body posture for long periods of time;
- avoid work where the tool transfers vibrations to the whole or part of the body;
- avoid exposing parts of the body to low temperatures including air flow from pneumatic tools;
- avoid, in particular, any combinations of the above conditions.

Table 7.1 Relationship between CTDs and occupational activities, from Kroemer, 1989

Disorder	Body activities	Typical job activities
Carpal tunnel syndrome	Repeated wrist flexion or extension, rapid wrist rotation, radial or ulnar deviation, forceful wrist motions and deviation, pressure with the palm, pinching	Buffing, grinding, polishing, sanding, assembly work, typing, keying, cashiering, playing musical instruments, surgery, packing, housekeeping, cooking, carpentry, brick laying, butchering, hand washing or scrubbing, hammering
Epicondylitis, tennis elbow	Radial wrist pronation with extension, forceful wrist extension, repeated supination and pronation, jerky throwing or impacting motions, forceful wrist extension with forearm pronation	Turning screws, small parts assembly, hammering, meat cutting, playing musical instruments, playing tennis, bowling
Neck tension syndrome	Prolonged static posture of neck/shoulder/arm, prolonged carrying of load on shoulder or in the hand	Belt conveyor assembly, typing, keying, small parts assembly, packing, load carrying in hand or on shoulder
Pronator teres syndrome	Rapid pronation of the forearm, forceful pronation, pronation with wrist flexion	Soldering, buffing, grinding, polishing, sanding
Radial tunnel syndrome	Repetitive wrist flexion with pronation or supination of the forearm	Use of hand tools
Shoulder tendonitis, rotator cuff syndrome	Shoulder abduction and flexion, arm extended, abducted, or flexed in the elbow more than 60 degrees, continuous elbow elevation, work with hand above shoulder, load carrying on shoulder, throwing object	Punch press operations, overhead assembly, overhead welding, overhead painting, overhead auto repair, belt conveyor assembly work, packing, storing, construction work, postal 'letter carrying', reaching, lifting

Tendonitis in the wrist	Forceful wrist extension and flexion, forceful ulnar deviation	Punch press operation, assembly work, wiring, packing, core making, use of pliers
Tenosynovitis, DeQuervain's syndrome ganglion	Wrist motions, forceful wrist extension and ulnar deviation while pushing or with supination, wrist flexion and extension with pressure at the palmar base, rapid rotations of the wrist	Buffing, grinding, polishing, sanding, punch press operation, sawing, cutting, surgery, butchering, use of pliers, 'turning' control such as on motorcycle, inserting screws in holes, forceful hand wringing
Thoracic outlet syndrome	Carrying heavy load in the hand, carrying load by shoulder strap, hyperextension of arm, shoulder flexion, prolonged restricted posture of upper body and arm, reaching overhead	Buffing, grinding, polishing, sanding, overhead assembly, overhead welding, overhead painting, overhead auto repair, typing, keying, cashiering, wiring, playing musical instruments, surgery, truck driving, stacking, material handling, postal 'letter carrying', carrying heavy loads with extended arms
Trigger finger	Repetitive finger flexion, sustained bending of the distal finger phalanx while more proximal phalanges are straight	Operating finger trigger, using hand tools where the handle opening is too large for the hand
Ulnar nerve entrapment, Guyon tunnel syndrome	Prolonged flexion and extension of the wrist, pressure on the hypothenar eminence, sustained elbow flexion with pressure on the ulnar groove	Playing musical instruments, carpentry, brick laying, use of pliers, soldering, hammering
White (or dead) finger syndrome, Raynaud's syndrome	Gripping of vibrating tool, using hand tool that hinders blood circulation	Chain sawing, jack hammering, use of vibrating tool, sanding, paint scraping, using tool too small for the hand, often in a cold environment

COST BENEFITS FROM THE APPLICATION OF ERGONOMICS

As has already been stated, one of the main obstacles to the widespread use of ergonomics in the workplace has been the failure to convince management of the cost benefits of introducing ergonomics. Of course, without the opportunity to carry out large-scale ergonomics studies in the first place, this problem is difficult to overcome. It is partly for this reason that the example described here to illustrate the benefits comes from Norway (Spilling, Eitrheim and Aaras, 1986). The study was carried out at Standard Telephone and Kabelfabrik A/S at Kongsvinger, a small rural town north of Oslo. The plant had a workforce of around 100, a majority of whom were women. The work involved the assembly and wiring of electromechanical components and racks. The impetus for the study was the progressive increase in the frequency of reported musculo-skeletal symptoms compared with other illnesses. Traditionally the work was performed at individual workstations with fixed working height. This meant that the operators had to adopt awkward working postures with excessive static workloads. In 1975 an extensive redesign of the workplaces took place which allowed greater flexibility of working posture and, in particular, allowed work to be performed while the operators were either sitting or standing. The main effect of the ergonomics intervention was to lower the long-term sickness attributable to musculo-skeletal disorders from an average of 5.3% of total production time before the change to 3.1% after the change. At the same time there was a 75% reduction in labour turnover in the years following the change. However, while this may have been in part due to improved workplace design it may also have been influenced by other factors such as changes in the general level of unemployment, although subsequent interviews with the operators strongly suggested that the reduction in turnover could be mainly attributable to the improved working conditions. Short-term sick leave remained the same after the change.

It is likely that only when it comes to considering the financial benefits of the ergonomics intervention programme, will a strong case be made for the benefits of the changes. Although there are always difficulties in deciding what to include in a cost-benefit analysis of this kind, Spilling *et al.* (1986) estimate that the value of the implementation over the period 1976 to 1988 was equivalent to £262 000. The investment in the ergonomics programme amounted to a meagre £31 000 while the savings in reduced recruitment costs, training costs, instructor salary costs, and in sick payments over the same period were estimated at £293 000. The project work itself has not been included in the investment costs, but according to the research team this was very small compared to the substantial savings. What should be emphasized

from this comprehensive long-term study is that the cost benefits
of implementing ergonomics cannot be assessed simply by using
traditional measures of productivity such as hourly or daily output
rates. Additionally, it should not be forgotten that there are hidden
benefits from ergonomics interventions which are difficult to express in
financial terms. For example, it is likely in the Norwegian study that
job satisfaction would have improved as well as the general quality of
both working and home life.

REFERENCES

Adams, J.A. (1989) *Human Factors Engineering*, Macmillan, New York, USA.
ANSI/HFS 100-1988 (1988) *American National Standard for Human Factors Engineering of Visual Display Terminal Workstations*, The Human Factors Society, Santa Monica, USA.
Astrand, P.O. and Rodahl, K. (1986) *Textbook of Work Physiology*, McGraw-Hill, New York, USA.
Boddy, D. and Buchanan, D.A. (1986) *Managing New Technology*, Basil Blackwell, Oxford, UK.
Booher, H.R. (1990) *MANPRINT. An Approach to Systems Integration*, Van Nostrand Reinhold, New York, USA.
BS 3044 (1990) Guide to Ergonomics Principles in the Design and Selection of Office Furniture, British Standards Institution, London, UK.
BS 4099 (1986) Colours of Indicator Lights, Push-buttons, Annunciators and Digital Readouts, British Standards Institution, London, UK.
BS 4467 (1991) Dimensions in Designing for Elderly People, British Standards Institution, London, UK.
BS 5304 (1988) Safety of Machinery, British Standards Institution, London, UK.
BS 5378 (1980) Safety Signs and Colours, British Standards Institution, London, UK.
BS 5940 (1980) Part 1: Specification for Design and Dimensions of Office Workstations, Desks, Tables and Chairs, British Standards Institution, London, UK.
BS 6841 (1987) Guide to Measurement and Evaluation of Human Exposure to Whole-Body Mechanical Vibration and Repeated Shock, British Standards Institution, London, UK.
BS 6842 (1987) Guide to Measurement and Evaluation to Vibration Transmitted to the Hand, British Standards Institution, London, UK.
BS 7179 (1990) Ergonomics of Design and Use of Visual Display Terminals (VDTs) in Offices, British Standards Institution, London, UK.
BS 7321 (1990) Body Measurements of Boys and Girls from Birth up to 16.9 Years, British Standards Institution, London, UK.
CIBSE (1978) *Environmental Criteria for Design*, Section A1, The Chartered Institution of Building Services Engineers, London, UK.
CIBSE (1994) *Code for Interior Lighting 1994*, The Chartered Institution of Building Services Engineers, London, UK.
Davis, L.E. and Taylor, J.C. (1979) *Design of Jobs*, 2nd edn, Goodyear, Santa Monica, USA.

DEF Stan 00-25 (1984–1992) Human Factors for Designers of Equipment, Ministry of Defence, Glasgow, Scotland.

Eason, K. (1988) *Information Technology and Organisational Change*, Taylor & Francis, London, UK.

Engels, J.A., Landeweerd, J.A. and Kant, Y. (1994) An OWAS-based analysis of nurses' working postures. *Ergonomics*, **37**(5), 900–19.

Griffin, M.J. (1990) *Handbook of Human Vibration*, Academic Press, London, UK.

Health and Safety at Work etc. Act 1974, HMSO, London, UK.

Health and Safety (Display Screen Equipment) Regulations 1992 (Statutory Instrument 1992, No. 2792), HMSO, London, UK.

Health and Safety Executive (1992) *Guidance on the Manual Handling Operations Regulations 1992*, HSE Books, Sudbury, UK.

Hickson, J. and Megaw, T. (1994) An example of job redesign in a large automotive plant, in *Contemporary Ergonomics 1994* (ed. S.A. Robertson), Taylor & Francis, London, pp. 400–5.

ISO 6385 (1991) Ergonomic Principles in the Design of Work Systems, International Organization for Standardization, Geneva, Switzerland.

ISO 9241 (1992) Ergonomic Requirements for Office Work with Visual Display Terminals (VDTs), International Organization for Standardization, Geneva, Switzerland.

Kant, I., Notermans, J.H.V. and Borm, P.J.A. (1990) Observations of working postures in garages using Ovako Working Posture Analysis System (OWAS) and consequent workload reduction recommendations. *Ergonomics*, **33**(2), 209–20.

Karhu, O., Kansi, P. and Kuorinka, I. (1977) Correcting working postures in industry: a practical method for analysis. *Applied Ergonomics*, **8**(4), 199–201.

Keyserling, W.M., Brouwer, M. and Silverstein, B.A. (1992) A checklist for evaluating ergonomic risk factors resulting from awkward postures of the legs, trunk and neck. *International Journal of Industrial Ergonomics*, **9**(4), 283–310.

Kivi, P. and Mattila, M. (1991) Analysis and improvement of work postures in the building industry: application of the computerised OWAS method. *Applied Ergonomics*, **22**(1), 43–8.

Kroemer, K.H.E. (1989) Cumulative trauma disorders: their recognition and ergonomics measures to avoid them. *Applied Ergonomics*, **20**(4), 274–80.

Kryter, K.D. (1985) *The Effects of Noise on Man*, 2nd edn, Academic Press, London, UK.

Kuorinka, I., Jonsson, B., Kilbom, A. *et al.* (1987) Standardised Nordic questionnaires for the analysis of musculoskeletal symptoms. *Applied Ergonomics*, **18**(3), 233–7.

McAtamney, L. and Corlett, E.N. (1993) RULA; a survey method for the investigation of work-related upper limb disorders. *Applied Ergonomics*, **24**(2), 91–9.

Management of Health and Safety at Work Regulations 1992 (Statutory Instrument 1992 No. 2051), HMSO, London, UK.

Manual Handling Operations Regulations 1992 (Statutory Instrument 1992 No. 2793), HMSO, London, UK.

Megaw, E.D. (1991) Ergonomics, trends and influences, in *International Review of Industrial and Organizational Psychology 1991*, **6** (eds C.L. Cooper and I.T. Robertson), Wiley, Chichester, pp. 109–48.

Mital, A., Nicholson, A.S. and Ayoub, M.M. (1993) *A Guide to Manual Materials Handling*, Taylor & Francis, London, UK.

Monk, T.H. and Folkard, S. (1992) *Making Shiftwork Tolerable*, Taylor & Francis, London, UK.

Murrell, H. (1965) *Men and Machines*, Methuen, London, UK.

NIOSH (1981) *A Work Practices Guide for Manual Lifting*, National Institute for Occupational Safety and Health, Cincinnati, Ohio, USA.

NIOSH (1991) *Revisions in NIOSH Guide to Manual Lifting*, National Institute for Occupational Safety and Health, Cincinnati, Ohio, USA.

Noise at Work Regulations 1989 (Statutory Instrument 1989 No. 1790), HMSO, London, UK.

Oborne, D.J. (1987) *Ergonomics at Work*, 2nd edn, Wiley, Chichester, UK.

Offices, Shops and Railway Premises Act 1963, HMSO, London, UK.

Parsons, K.C. (1993) *Human Thermal Environments*, Taylor and Francis, London, UK.

Perrow, C. (1984) *Normal Accidents: Living with High-risk Technologies*, Basic Books, New York, USA.

Personal Protective Equipment at Work Regulations 1992 (Statutory Instrument 1992, No. 2966), HMSO, London, UK.

Pheasant, S. (1986) *Bodyspace: Anthropometry, Ergonomics and Design*, Taylor and Francis, London, UK.

Pheasant, S. (1991) *Ergonomics, Work and Health*, Macmillan, Basingstoke, UK.

Provision and Use of Work Equipment Regulations 1992 (Statutory Instrument 1992, No. 2932), HMSO, London, UK.

Putz-Anderson, V. (ed.) (1988) *Cumulative Trauma Disorders. A Manual for Musculoskeletal Diseases of the Upper Limbs*, Taylor & Francis, London, UK.

Rubinstein, E. and Mason, A.F. (1979) The accident that shouldn't have happened: an analysis of Three Mile Island. *IEEE Spectrum*, **16**, 33–57.

Salvendy, G. and Karwowski, W. (eds) (1994) *Design of Work and Development of Personnel in Advanced Manufacturing*, Wiley, New York, USA.

Sanders, M.S. and McCormick, E.J. (1992) *Human Factors in Engineering and Design*, 7th edn, McGraw-Hill, New York, USA.

Spilling, S., Eitrheim, J. and Aaras A. (1986) Cost-benefit analysis of work environment investment at STK's telephone plant at Kongsvinger, in *The Ergonomics of Working Postures* (ed. E.N. Corlett, J. Wilson and I. Manenica), Taylor & Francis, London, UK, pp. 380–97.

Stubbs, D. and Buckle, P. (1991) The benefits of ergonomics intervention with particular reference to physical strain, in *Towards Human Work* (ed. M. Kumashiro and E.D. Megaw), Taylor & Francis, London, UK, pp. 108–14.

Swezey, R.W. and Salas, E. (1992) *Teams: Their Training and Performance*, Ablex, Norwood New Jersey, USA.

Waters, T.R., Putz-Anderson, V., Garg, A. and Fine, L.J. (1993) Revised NIOSH equation for the design and evaluation of manual lifting tasks. *Ergonomics*, **36**(7), 749–76.

Wilson, J.R. and Corlett, E.N. (eds) (1990) *Evaluation of Human Work: A Practical Methodology*, Taylor and Francis, London, UK.

Woodson, W.E., Tillman, B. and Tillman, P. (1992) *Human Factors Design Handbook*, 2nd edn, McGraw-Hill, New York, USA.

Workplace (Health, Safety and Welfare) Regulations 1992 (Statutory Instrument 1992, No. 3004), HMSO, London, UK.

Occupational hygiene   8

Steven Bailey

MODERN OCCUPATIONAL HYGIENE PRACTICE

Once upon a time occupational hygiene was about preventing:

- acute lead poisoning
- coal miners' pneumoconiosis
- silicosis in the cutlery industry
- asbestos diseases in manufacturing and construction
- byssinosis in the cotton industry
- kidney damage from cadmium poisoning
- bladder cancer in dyestuffs and rubber factories.

It is testimony to the work of occupational hygienists (and others) that most of these occupational diseases no longer present significant problems in advanced countries. In some cases the offending substances have been replaced by less toxic ones, in others they are now used in a controlled way. In every instance the cause of the problem is now understood and preventive or protective measures are available. Only asbestos continues to show increasing incidence rates because of the long lead time (20–50 years) before the development of disease: actual conditions in the industry have long since been improved.

This should not give rise to complacency. The march of technology constantly brings forwards new substances and processes which may prove to be catastrophically harmful. Examples like the discovery of hepatic angiosarcoma from vinyl chloride monomer in 1974 emphasize the importance of constant vigilance. Such is the pace and variety of innovation that never has the opportunity for calamity been greater.

And yet for the most part the modern hygienist does not deal on a daily basis with such headline-making concerns. Indeed the insidious nature of occupational disease means that it rarely reaches the news.

- Skin contact with chemicals has been estimated to produce 80 000 cases a year of occupational dermatitis in the UK alone, many of them disabling and with a very poor prognosis of recovery.
- Some 500 cases a year of occupational asthma are diagnosed through chest physicians (Health and Safety Commission, 1992).
- Around a million people in the UK are still exposed to levels of noise which could damage their hearing.
- In total, the Health and Safety Executive estimates that 750 000 workers in the UK had time off for work related illness in 1989–90. Of all GP consultations by working age patients, 7% were work related (OHR Feature, 1994).

Occupational disease may not be dramatic but it blights many lives and in some cases ends them. So why is it allowed to continue?

The first reason is that proving cause and effect can be difficult. Long response times, the lack of good exposure or morbidity data and the mobility of the workforce all complicate the issue. In many cases experts don't even agree whether there is a problem or not. Examples include the neurological effects of solvent exposure, sick building syndrome, and the effects of low-level lead exposure on intelligence and behaviour.

Apathy is the second reason. Even where the risks are established beyond reasonable doubt, employers and employees continue to ignore them. As long ago as 1713, Ramazzini enunciated the principle that to achieve control of the working environment you must eliminate interference from the worker. Despite mechanization and automation this remains the crux of the problem. Training and management systems are perhaps even more important than before as the best available technology of control increasingly proves inadequate.

It is the task of the modern hygienist to recognize, evaluate and where necessary control such risks. In the words of the Institute of Occupational Hygienists:

> Occupational hygiene is the application of scientific, technological and managerial principles for the protection of health by the prevention or reduction of risks to health from chemical, biological or physical agents whether the risks are to people at the workplace or outside it.
>
> IOH, 1993

THE PROBLEM WITH OELS

DEVELOPMENT OF OELS

The ability to measure the exposure of employees to hazardous agents in the air of the workplace is one of the key skills of the hygienist.

Indeed, much of modern occupational hygiene practice is predicated on it. As instrumentation has developed measurement has become progressively easier and the results more reliable. Moreover the results can now be interpreted against a comprehensive set of Occupational Exposure Limits (OELs) (HSE, 1994) with supporting documentation (HSE, 1993). Paradoxically, this has led to a false sense of security and to the belief that controlling environments to the OEL will eliminate problems.

OELs originated in the USA as guidelines for professionals to be applied with understanding and circumspection. The current American listing of Threshold Limit Values still clings to this view (ACGIH, 1993). Government agencies such as OSHA, however, have sought to use OELs as compliance testing tools. Legislators and the general public often see OELs as a magic solution to hygiene problems. It appears that industry has only to stay below the prescribed numbers – which can easily be tested – and everything will be all right. Conversely, exceeding the OEL is seen as presenting serious and imminent danger. These simplistic notions rely on a failure to appreciate the scientific basis of the standards.

Respiratory sensitizers provide one simple example of why the regulatory OEL approach does not work: attacks of asthma can be triggered in sensitized individuals by minute amounts of material, well below the OEL. Problems also arise with materials (including many organic solvents) which can be absorbed through the skin, where high exposures may arise through skin contact even though airborne levels are controlled.

Measurement of atmospheric exposure is necessary as a check on the performance of control measures, but compliance with the OEL by itself is insufficient to protect workers. It has to be one element of a package. To understand fully the limitations (and the correct use) of OELs it is necessary to look more closely at the technical principles which underlie them.

EXPOSURE MEASUREMENT

The amount of a contaminant in the air of a workplace is not static. It varies with time and with location according to such factors as the type of work being carried out, the throughput, the behaviour of the employees and climatic conditions. Thus the simple question 'What is the concentration in the workplace air?' does not have a simple answer. The answer has to be qualified by the circumstances of the measurements and the statistical variability of the results.

This would not be important if the statistical variation were small (say, a few per cent) and if the factors causing the variation were easily identified and controlled. In practice the variations can span orders of magnitude and the determining factors are elusive. The problem has been known to practising hygienists for a long time (King, 1980; Higgins, 1982; Bailey and Miles, 1984), though only recently has it been thoroughly explored by theoreticians (Rappaport, 1991; Kromhout, Symanski and Rappaport, 1993). Most legislators seem to remain blissfully unaware of the implications when we come to measure the airborne concentration to which a worker is exposed.

Firstly, it means that the positioning of the sampler is crucial. A sampler fixed near to the worker (a 'static' sample) will commonly give results which differ by a factor of 2–10 from those of a sampler actually attached to the worker (a 'personal' sample). Consequently, any data obtained from static samples should be discounted in setting or testing compliance with an OEL. The impending revision of the UK standard for cotton dust, which was traditionally based on static sampling, illustrates how important this can be (Ogden *et al.*, 1993).

Even simultaneous paired personal samples on a single worker show a range of up to 3:1. These differences are often random, depending on invisible and unpredictable air currents. Some systematic effects also occur. For example, when a worker is handling a toxic powder, dust levels near his or her nose or mouth are likely to be lower than levels at the lapel. Traditional personal sampling equipment is lapel mounted and so overestimates exposure in such situations. The need for a true breathing zone sampler has been recognized for some time (Bloor, Eardley and Dinsdale, 1968; Allen, Bellinger and Higgins, 1981).

It also follows that the number of samples needed to make valid judgements is large, because the extent of random fluctuations has to be assessed and allowed for in estimating the true exposure. Assuming a lognormal distribution of data with a geometric standard deviation of 2.0 (a common situation in a well-controlled environment), it can be calculated that 40 samples are needed to estimate the mean exposure to within ±25%. Thus taking a handful of samples is not sufficient either to provide a basis for an OEL or to test compliance.

These inherent difficulties are compounded by the fact that sampling equipment is imperfect and there are large bias errors between different types of sampler, depending on geometry, orientation, flow patterns and electrostatic effects (Allen, 1983).

LIMIT SETTING

OELs fall into two types. Health-based limits are, essentially, safe levels. They take no account of the cost or practicability of achieving those levels. In the UK they are represented by Occupational Exposure Standards and in Europe by Indicative Limit Values. The second category of OELs might be called socioeconomic limits. They entail a balance of risk against cost and feasibility, with due allowance made for uncertainties in the risk estimates. They do not purport to be safe levels, rather they are the upper limits of acceptability. Maximum Exposure Limits are of this kind. Clearly the two types of limit must be set by different processes: one is a purely scientific measure whilst the other is a political judgement. The validity of either though depends on having good data available to underpin the limit setting process.

For a health-based limit, the data requirements are primarily toxicological and epidemiological. The toxicology is usually difficult to interpret because of interspecies differences, inappropriate dose levels, etc. Human experience is therefore preferable when it is available. Here we encounter the well-known problems of confounding factors and poorly matched control groups, but it is the characterization of exposure that is often the weakest link in epidemiological studies. Frequently such studies fail to specify the sampling equipment used or the strategy adopted. This precludes proper comparison of different studies and makes it impossible to analyse the effect of using different equipment or strategies for compliance testing.

One extreme, but not isolated, example of how sampling strategy can affect OELs is kaolin dust. Here the proposed Occupational Exposure Standard of $2.5\,mg\,m^{-3}$ is set on the basis of the long-term exposure level (i.e. the average exposure) that produced no effect in the study population. But compliance is tested on the basis that no 8-hour sample should exceed the OEL. Assuming a typical spread of sampling results, the average (long-term) exposure level in the industry will have to be held to about one-quarter of the limit in order to comply on individual 8-hour samples. Scientifically, the limit should have been set at a value (perhaps) four times higher to be consistent with the epidemiology.

For socioeconomic limits the legislators also need good data on current exposure levels and an assessment of how far exposures can be reduced at what cost. This fundamental hygiene information is almost never available. Thus such limits are usually negotiated compromises with neither side actually understanding the full implications of what has been agreed.

COMPLIANCE TESTING AND ENFORCEMENT

To test compliance properly requires a statistically designed sampling protocol and a large number of samples (Dewell, 1989). Commonly this demands resources which are not available or which could be put more productively to other uses. The alternative strategy is to take only a small number of samples and compare each value obtained individually with the OEL. When an occasional value exceeds the OEL, repeating the test will usually produce a lower result purely by chance and so will justify inaction. This is cheating. Individual sample results that are below the OEL do not prove compliance on an ongoing basis.

Thus the consequence of legally enforceable OELs is that the hygienist has to choose between wasting resources on unproductive statistical sampling or adopting a sampling regime that he or she knows to be dishonest.

Inspectors trying to enforce OELs often face a similar dilemma. Only when the OEL is grossly exceeded so that virtually every individual sample exceeds the limit is the infringement proven. It is not surprising then that in most countries action is rarely taken on the basis of high air sampling results alone. When OELs are cited, it is usually as a convenient prop to support the inspector's pre-judged diagnosis that control measures are inadequate.

This is not necessarily a bad thing. Rigid enforcement of OELs using a statistical protocol (as has been done in the USA) can lead to excessive effort being devoted to sampling and administration at the expense of preventive measures. For the moment the element of judgement is retained in Europe, which was always the hallmark of professional use of OELs. They continue to be a valuable investigative tool for the hygienist, so long as they do not become political footballs.

Unfortunately it means that we also have to look elsewhere for ways of protecting workers.

CULTURE

THE IMPORTANCE OF CULTURE

The importance of management's attitude in achieving control of the working environment is well recognized. It has become common to talk about developing a 'safety culture'. Health and safety should form part of the daily running of the organization, not be a bolt-on extra.

Organizations, however, are not blank sheets of paper. They already have cultures. A simple classification identifies four primary types: power, role, task and person cultures (Handy, 1985). Each has a different management style, a different technique for getting the best out of people. None is necessarily better than the others, but the culture has to be appropriate to the organization's purpose and scale. It would be inappropriate to manage a small advertising agency the same way as a large insurance company, or to run a car repair shop like a university. Briefly the four cultural types may be summarized as follows.

The power culture

Typified by many small owner-managed businesses, the power culture is controlled by the person in the centre. Communication tends to be on a need-to-know basis and even minor decisions require authorization. Paperwork systems are often absent, with all key information held in the boss's head. There are no committees and few meetings.

Such companies can be flexible, responsive to the market and often engender in their employees a great deal of pride. To work there, however, you have to fit into the culture. Any challenge is likely to be put down ruthlessly.

Power cultures find it difficult to grow beyond 10–20 people as the power-source becomes overstretched. Entrepreneurs will often sell their business and leave rather than submit to the culture change demanded by growth. Where power cultures survive into large businesses it is usually by spawning subsidiary businesses which are managed by a loyal ally of the power source.

The role culture

Power in the role culture comes from position. Job descriptions are more important than the individual who fills the post. Organizational structures and formal procedures dictate who makes decisions and how things get done. Hierarchy is all important, and will be very evident in committee meetings, budgets and authority to act.

Many large companies (in oil, insurance, banking, etc.) and most government departments are of this type. They are the classic bureaucracies. This should not be interpreted negatively as such organizations have great strengths. They are predictable and secure. Economies of scale are practicable. They are able to produce a high quality product consistently year after year, even though individuals may leave. They reward achievement of standards, provide routes for career progression and individuals can develop deep specializations.

But role cultures suffer when change is needed. Their whole structure is designed to protect the status quo and will resist innovation. They do not respond quickly to changes in their environment. People who want more control over their jobs find role culture frustrating.

The task culture

Sometimes referred to as 'democratic', the task culture is a modern development. It is devoted to getting the job done, quickly and efficiently, in a changing environment. People work in informal teams, which may be formed for specific projects and disbanded as soon as they are finished. There are often no job descriptions and no clear hierarchy. Even budgets and authority levels may be unclear. Power is based on expertise and performance. Skills tend to be broad rather than deep, because versatility is the prime requirement. To an outsider it can appear chaotic, but this permits the flexibility needed for rapid change.

Consultancies often work this way; so do industries where the product lifetime is short making innovation paramount, and service departments (such as marketing) which interface with the customer. They are fast, exciting places to work in, but are not for the insecure. They are difficult organizations to manage as decisions have to be made by consensus, not imposed. Trust is high, but conflict can quickly develop. Communication is by face-to-face discussion. Written procedures, if they are ever drafted, are usually obsolete before they are finalized.

The person culture

Few organizations have this type of culture. Rather it represents the perspective of some individuals within an organization who see their role as more important than the performance of the organization overall. Professors in universities and hospital consultants epitomize these characteristics. They are tolerated by the organization because the organization needs their abilities, but they regard the organization simply as somewhere to do their own thing and show little allegiance.

Managing such people is difficult. Organizational rules and policies are treated with disdain unless they are developed by mutual consent. Often the position of such people will be protected by a contract of tenure. Generally only role culture organizations will accept this sort of cultural elitism in their midst.

NATIONAL CULTURE

Onto these organizational cultures we must superimpose the effect of national culture. Mole (1993) has analysed the impact of different national cultures within the European Union on the way companies are managed in each country. The differences are startling. Management systems which would be welcomed in one country are rejected as burdensome in another or inadequate in a third.

These characteristic ways of operating must be taken into account if any occupational hygiene initiative is to be successful. Clearly, a 'health and safety culture' will have to take different forms in different companies if it is to be accepted and integrated within an organization's own philosophy and systems. Current trends in EC driven legislation and HSE guidance in the UK promote a role culture approach to health and safety. They require defined responsibilities, written procedures, audits, etc. These systems will be readily recognized and adopted by organizations which have role cultures. To many small and medium-sized enterprises they will be completely alien. Small and medium enterprises (SMEs) would have to change their entire business culture in order to adapt.

PRESSURES FOR CULTURAL CHANGE

Cultures evolve over time. The culture of our own society is changing quite naturally and this is exerting pressure on the way that companies are managed.

Increasing international exchange of information and the growth of multinational companies have led to pressures for harmonization. National cultures have begun adapting in response. This is most obvious in the case of the European Union with its central Directives and Regulations.

European legislation is more prescriptive than the UK style of the last 20 years. The Robens report (1972) initiated a new framework of legislation in the UK through the Health and Safety at Work Act 1974. Section 2.1 of the Act puts the onus on employers to protect the safety and health of their employees so far as is reasonably practicable but leaves the mechanism open for the employers to choose. The new EC style framework Directive (89/391/EEC) and the individual directives flowing from it are more specific in a number of areas. This has created an eruption of new legislation in the UK, much of it geared to role culture doctrines.

One of the most visible changes has been the requirement for formal risk assessments of all work activities (regulation 3 of the Management of Health and Safety at Work Regulations 1992.) Risk assessment has always been the cornerstone of the UK approach to occupational hygiene: in legal terms it underlies the concept of reasonable practicability which is at the centre of UK health and safety law. But hitherto it has always been implicit; now as a result of European legislation it is explicit. For many companies (and many professionals) this implies a change in culture much more than a change in standards.

The pressure has come from other quarters too. Part of the drive for systems and systematic control has come from quality assurance (Deacon, 1994). BS 5750 the quality standard and its European and international equivalents, the EN 29000 and ISO 9000 series, are premised on the need to prove what was done and why. Everything must be documented. Some large companies have embraced the quality systems approach themselves and then imposed it on their smaller suppliers. The scene is now set for a similar transformation in health and safety. Indeed the British Standard (BS 8750) is already under development.

Ironically these pressures arise at a time when the pace of technological change is pushing society towards smaller and more flexible enterprises. SMEs represent a high proportion of the workforce.

CULTURE IN SMES

The role culture fits well with many established large organizations. Control is achieved though bureaucracy. It is less satisfactory for SMEs.

Most entrepreneurs start a business because they want the freedom and opportunities it offers and have the relevant technical skills to contribute. They already feel burdened with tax law, insurances, contract law, employment law and so on. Now they see a growing threat from health and safety legislation. It is not just that the volume of administration is tedious or demanding. Small businesses thrive on flexibility, innovation and verbal communication and can be stifled by paperwork systems that might be essential in a larger company. Rigid rules and record keeping conflict with the natural culture of most SMEs.

Finding ways of accommodating SMEs within the new framework without strangling them is one of the great challenges to occupational hygiene. Failure to allow for cultural variety will result in the imposition of a system that is doomed from the outset as it is tolerated rather than owned by management. An alternative approach must be found.

ACHIEVING A SAFETY CULTURE

The modern trend, now enshrined in UK and EC legislation, is to use management systems to provide the necessary element of control over health risks at work. This systems approach can be very effective where the culture of the organization is appropriate and the necessary driving force is present.

Case Study 1 illustrates the use of a classic management systems approach to an occupational hygiene problem. Whilst undeniably successful it suffered from shortcomings that are typical of many, otherwise effective, management systems:

- they can be bureaucratic and burdensome;
- they are more effective at maintaining the status quo than at dealing with change;
- the belief that the system provides the control can obscure the real purpose of the exercise. The importance of vigilance may be forgotten.

CASE STUDY 1

A large manufacturing organization introduced a Legionella management system after experiencing an outbreak. In sequence they:

- retained a consultant to audit their sites and review existing practices;
- created an internal code of practice which provided for
  - named staff to be responsible for Legionella control
  - policies on purchase and installation of plant
  - notification of new and changed water systems
  - regular cleaning, treatment and maintenance of relevant plant
  - regular inspection and testing of plant as appropriate
  - documentation of all actions and results in a quality assured format
  - internal and external audits of performance and an annual review of the code
- staff trained staff in the hazards of Legionella and the operation of the code;
- implemented the code.

The successful outcome was to reduce to a very low level the likelihood of a further outbreak of Legionnaire's disease. After two years the programme was still running satisfactorily. Key factors in the success of the programme were identified as:

- the commitment of senior management, resulting from their earlier experience which afforded a high priority to the programme;
- the appointment of competent and committed staff to oversee the programme, including a professional administrator to issue the necessary forms and keep the records;
- the use of an external consultant to monitor the programme and chase progress.

Nonetheless, some difficulties were experienced:

- paperwork was onerous and demanded considerable resource;
- new and changed plant was not consistently notified and was discovered after the event. Refresher training had to be given to those responsible.

It would have been inconceivable to introduce such a system into most small companies. Even if they were able to afford it, it is unlikely that management would have the commitment to keep it running. From choice, most responsible small companies would have opted for a much simpler and less formal system.

Systems alone do not generate an ongoing commitment. Long-term protection is predicated on creating and sustaining awareness of the hazard and the need for controls. Awareness alone is not always sufficient to prompt and maintain appropriate actions, but in combination with systems, awareness holds the key.

Awareness may come from education (other people's experience suitably presented) or personal experience or both. Of course, personal experience is gained after the event and is clearly an unsatisfactory premise for developing awareness or protecting health and safety. Education is thus the starting point for fostering awareness.

CASE STUDY 2

A major manufacturing organization attempted to implement the COSHH Regulations when they were first introduced. The initial programme included significant investment in the preparation of an assessment protocol and the training of assessors. A review of the position three years later found that:

- most assessors had changed jobs and new ones had not been trained;
- there was no real commitment to COSHH at senior management level;
- the level of awareness at supervisory and shop floor levels was very low;
- few of the initial assessments had been implemented.

Historically, management's response to these findings would probably have been to introduce further procedural controls. At this time, however, the company was engaged in a long-term programme of cultural change. Management's new response was to undertake an extensive programme of employee awareness and skills training. Within months this had the effect of sharply raising consciousness about the hazards of chemicals. It is now noticeable that many employees refer to COSHH considerations in their everyday work. This new commitment must inevitably lead to improved protection from chemical hazards.

There is a close parallel here with the introduction of the quality standard BS 5750, which has been heavily criticized for similar reasons. It relies on management systems to achieve quality and strives for consistency and proof of performance. But it does not question whether the actual standard of quality needs improvement and it frequently fails to generate real commitment. The complementary concept of Total Quality Management seeks to overcome this by building a cultural commitment to quality, just as many organizations are now trying to build safety cultures.

The greater the degree to which employees can be trusted to take care of their own safety the less need there is for formal management systems. That is not to say that formal systems become unnecessary, rather that there is a balance to be struck. There is an inverse relationship between the extent to which people are educated to risks and the degree of supervision and record keeping necessary. Case Study 2 illustrates the advantage of the cultural approach over simple administrative systems.

Thus education underpins management systems. It enables administrative requirements to be reduced to a minimum and allows the management system to be matched to the culture of the organization. It also ensures that the system does not fail through lack of interest. Indeed, once safety awareness becomes part of the organizational culture it becomes self-sustaining.

THE MANAGEMENT ROLE OF THE HYGIENIST

THE PRESSURES FOR CHANGE

Traditionally most hygienists have been scientists, able to investigate health hazards and recommend process or engineering solutions. It will already be clear that to be effective a hygienist must now be able to develop and administer a management system, and to deliver safety education.

Traditionally, again, the skills required by a hygienist were quite different to those of a safety officer. The safety officer's role was often as a policeman, enforcing clear-cut rules on behaviour, machinery guarding, etc. The hygienist's skills were rooted in the ability to measure things that could not be seen and to predict long-term consequences. But huge changes have occurred in the safety profession over the last 10 years. Risk assessment has now formally entered the field and the safety professional is as involved in predicting future events as is the hygienist. Both have a major interest in management systems and employee education programmes. Topical subjects like manual handling and display screens cross the boundaries and the distinction has blurred. Both specialists are now health and safety professionals; their technical skills overlap and differ only in emphasis not in kind.

The changes do not stop there. With the advent of the Environmental Protection Act 1990, industry suddenly needed people who could measure and predict what was happening to the environment. Risk assessment became an integral part of environmental legislation, being a requirement for authorization under the Act. This type of work is in fact a natural extension of the hygienist's role. Occupational hygiene can be thought of as the study of concentrated environmental pollution in the workplace. Many of the assessment techniques used by hygienists are directly transferable to the external environment. What is more the actions recommended by hygienists to protect workers (e.g. exhaust ventilation) often impact on the external environment so an integrated approach is highly desirable. This interaction has been recognized in the EC Regulations on new and existing substances which require industry to submit data on both workplace and environmental hazards at the same time.

So at a time when economic constraints have limited recruitment, many health and safety practitioners have found their role extended to environment. This doesn't only imply a change in the volume of work, it triggers a fresh approach. Increasingly we will see a new breed of health, safety and environmental managers. While competent in the basics of measurement and engineering control their primary attributes will be managerial skills: communication, persuasion, leadership and delegation. They will occupy more senior positions in the company hierarchy and will require an understanding of business (including marketing and finance) so that they can contribute directly to high level decisions.

AUDITING

An audit is a systematic critical examination of management and/or technical systems to assess whether they meet set standards. Usually the objectives fall into one of two broad categories:

- to assess liability, e.g. pre-acquisition or pre-disposal;
- to assess compliance with legislation or company policies.

By conducting audits on a regular basis it is possible to detect improvements in performance that should be congratulated or deterioration before it is reflected in occupational disease statistics. Thus they provide a useful management tool.

There are a number of proprietary auditing systems available in health and safety, which provide prepared questions and often incorporate some sort of scoring system. The majority of these ready-made systems are quite weak on occupational hygiene aspects as opposed to physical safety and the hygienist may well need to tailor-make an audit protocol. However, the precise questions asked are less important than the basic approach, which will nearly always be the same.

Pre-visit

The company or site should be informed of the audit, its format, scope and objectives. In the case of consultant hygienists it is very important that these details are agreed with the client in advance. A liaison person should be appointed on site.

Generally it is preferable to have at least two people, with different backgrounds, in the audit team. In some cases more may be needed to provide the range of expertise required. A lead auditor should be appointed to act as the focal point for liaison with the company and to ensure that the audit is fully coordinated.

The company will then be asked to provide background information for study prior to the visit. Depending on the circumstances, this might include the health and safety policy, plans of the site, process flowcharts, copies of substance inventories, COSHH assessments, etc.

Opening meeting

It is essential to meet with senior managers at the start of the audit, to introduce the auditors and to enlist the managers' cooperation. At the same time it is useful to get their views on any particular matters that should be addressed and to assess their overall awareness of the issues. Typically this should take about 30 minutes. Timings of key meetings can be arranged at the end of the session.

Familiarization tour

Immediately after the opening meeting the auditors will want to tour the site to get their bearings and to plan time allocations. A knowledgeable guide (such as the site maintenance engineer or chemist) will prove invaluable.

Interviews and inspections

The bulk of the audit will consist of interviews with key staff, inspection of records and procedures, and in some cases physical examination of the plant.

Typically the auditors will want to see the plant manager, engineer, chemist, safety and medical officers and union safety representatives. In addition a sample of department managers and shop floor employees should be quizzed, generally on an informal basis while touring the plant.

It is not essential to follow a fixed list of questions. Well-structured open questions built around a checklist of key subjects will usually elicit the necessary information as completely as (and more quickly than) a questionnaire. As a starting point though, the Workwell audit system used in Ontario provides a good framework of questions covering the management of health and safety, viz. policies and procedures, programme development, implementation, promotion and communication.

Interviews should always be conducted in confidence and comments made should not be reported without permission. However, a full record of all discussions should be kept by the auditors for reference. It is useful to prepare standard record sheets for interviews and to develop a shorthand notation to identify follow-up actions required (Greeno, Hedstrom and Diberto, 1988).

A fundamental principle of auditing is that all information gained from interviews must be verified. This may involve asking to see the written records or policy statement, or physically checking the plant. Hearsay evidence can be a valuable prompt to uncover problems, but should always be cross-checked with those directly concerned.

Physical inspection of the plant may be needed to ensure that the company has taken all hazards into account and that control measures are working correctly. Documentation alone rarely gives an adequate picture of housekeeping, personal hygiene or maintenance standards. An inspection tour also provides the opportunity to question employees more naturally than in a formal interview.

Exit meeting

The exit meeting normally involves the same group of people as the opening meeting. It provides a chance for the auditors to thank everyone for participating and to explain the arrangements for reporting. Most importantly though, it gives some immediate feedback on the preliminary findings of the audit and smoothes the way for any criticisms to be made in the report. If the audit team has got a basic point badly wrong it should become evident, and be resolved at this stage.

Report

Audit reports always need an Executive Summary and an Action Plan to ensure that the main conclusions are easy to find and will be read. Some auditors like to express the results as numerical scores which can then be compared with other sites or monitored over time. Whether this quantitative approach finds favour depends on the culture of the company more than on any absoulte merit.

Reports should generally be submitted in draft to allow the company to point out any errors of fact before they are finalized. This avoids any acrimony caused by petty mistakes and helps to win management's commitment to implementation.

RISK ASSESSMENT AS AN OPPORTUNITY

The requirement for risk assessment of all work activities under the Management of Health and Safety at Work Regulations 1992 implies new and potentially burdensome duties for employers. SMEs in particular have expressed their concern. In many cases they do not understand the requirements, feel overwhelmed by the size of the task, lack the specific knowledge or skills required and are unable to judge the level of risks accurately.

At the same time risk assessment provides an opportunity to rationalize the use of resources and streamline existing procedures. Risk assessment can be used constructively to protect the health and safety of people at work through cost-effective management. Hygienists must make sure that this opportunity is grasped.

The procedure for carrying out a risk assessment can be divided into five stages as follows.

(i) Identify the hazards present

A hazard is a source of potential harm. For example, it may be an energy supply, a piece of equipment, a harmful substance or simply a situation. The presence of a hazard does not necessarily imply that harm is likely to occur in practice, but the identification of the hazard is a necessary first step in risk assessment.

(ii) Evaluate the risk they present

Risk denotes the likelihood of harm occurring under particular circumstances. For example, a cup of pure water presents little risk but a reservoir containing 100 million gallons poses an altogether different problem. In any particular situation we need to weight up the **risk factors**, i.e. the circumstances which make a particular event or outcome more or less likely to occur in practice. Typical risk factors for chemical hazards include the quantity used, duration of exposure, degree of skin contact, volatility or dustability of the material, etc. Each risk factor will contribute to our judgement of the risk occurring in practice. Inevitably this judgement will vary somewhat from one assessor to another but it forms a basis for deciding the priority to be given to control measures.

(iii) Decide the precautions necessary

It may be that legal requirements or company rules leave no choice as to the precautions to be taken. If there is a choice, the important question to answer is 'Will the precautions contemplated eliminate or minimize the risk?'

(iv) Record the findings if they are significant

It is desirable to limit record keeping to a minimum in order to avoid cumbersome and unworkable demands on assessors. Unless this is made a conscious policy, records are likely to proliferate. Detailed records should not be justified on the grounds that they may one day prove useful to defend the company. The only essential information is that needed to show how a decision was reached, so that the decision can be verified and the work need not be repeated unless conditions change.

For routine jobs, records are best held in the form of standard procedures for the work to be carried out, such as are commonly produced for quality assurance purposes. A statement of risks and the precautions to be taken can be added to existing procedures with minimal difficulty and without creating a new paperwork system.

Standard operating procedures are less satisfactory in situations where the work is non-repetitive and decisions have to be made on the spot. In such cases a simple checklist approach will often suffice. The person conducting the work fills in the checklist and files it as a record. This commonsense procedure depends on giving employees a high standard of training and supervising them effectively. If this cannot be done for any reason then a more rigid system of documentation is likely to be necessary.

(v) Set priorities for action

Proper discrimination of high risks is a big factor in focusing expenditure and effort. The most common mistake is to 'play safe' by assuming that all hazards need control, without assessing the likelihood of harm occurring.

This causes needless expenditure and distracts attention from the real issues. In most situations, once the risk has been evaluated, it will be obvious what priority should be given to action. A simple 'high, medium or low' system will often suffice. If there are a large number of situations to consider, though, it may help to use a more formal technique for setting priorities. One way of doing this is to use a matrix such as that in Table 8.1.

The classification is a matter for judgement and company policy, but simple guidelines can be helpful. For instance:

Table 8.1 Setting priorities

Likelihood (risk)	Severity of harm (hazard)		
	Minor	Moderate	Major
Very unlikely	Trivial	Tolerable	Moderate
Unlikely	Tolerable	Moderate	High
Likely	Moderate	High	Extreme

Trivial	– no action required
Tolerable	– maintain existing controls
	– improve if easy/cheap
Moderate	– reduce risk further
	– action within months
High	– improve substantially
	– action within weeks
Extreme	– stop immediately

Some people prefer to use more categories to give better discrimination, but the judgement required becomes correspondingly more difficult. Some companies prefer to put numbers on the categories and derive a risk score. This is a matter of culture and preference rather than technical advantage. It is also possible to build in a factor to allow explicitly for the number of people who may be affected.

There is no doubt that the new requirement to carry out risk assessment will lead to some additional work for managers and will necessitate improved training and more record keeping. However, if applied properly it will provide the opportunity to focus effort on those risks which are important and this will enable good managements to apply their resources more cost effectively. Competent judgement of risk levels is therefore crucial.

Training people to be competent in risk assessment is an expensive business. This cost, however, must be seen in the context of failure to use competent assessors. Aside from the obvious problems caused by inadequate assessment and therefore ineffective control (injury and prosecution) serious problems can be caused by over-cautious assessments. It is unfortunately common to see wasted expenditure and burdensome procedures being introduced because of the failure to assess risk accurately. Many untrained assessors do not adequately differentiate between hazard and risk and thus apply excessive controls in low risk situations. This leads to a loss of perspective where all hazards are treated the same.

COMPETENCY OF HYGIENISTS

Regulation 6(1) of the Management of Health and Safety at Work Regulations 1992 requires that every employer shall appoint one or more competent persons to assist him or her. Competent is defined as having such training, experience, knowledge and other qualities as are necessary.

Thus the person carrying out risk assessments must have the technical competence to recognize hazards, judge the level of risk (knowing when measurements are needed) and identify appropriate controls. Likewise a person taking air samples must be able to select the correct equipment and devise an appropriate sampling strategy. Other abilities are necessary to design a local exhaust system, choose appropriate personal protective equipment, etc. These are some of the traditional technical skills of the occupational hygienist, but it will not always be necessary to engage a professional hygienist to handle simple situations.

In practical terms the easiest way for an employer to ensure that the right skills are available is for the person to hold or obtain appropriate qualifications. The qualification which is most widely applicable is the certificate examination of the National Examining Board in Occupational Safety and Health (NEBOSH). This is an introductory qualification denoting awareness of health and safety risks in a wide range of situations. It can be taken either as a short course or by open learning, and is suitable for managers with a broad responsibility for health and safety. Where the degree of risk is higher or the complexity of the operations is greater, it may be advisable for the assessor to hold the NEBOSH Diploma which is the professional qualification in health and safety.

If the risks arise mainly from environmental workplace hazards such as chemicals or noise then a more specific qualification is an advantage. The preliminary certificates of the British Examining Board in Occupational Hygiene (BEBOH) provide specific training and test competence in these areas. They are suitable for technicians who are required to take air samples or conduct noise surveys, or to carry out basic COSHH assessments. From 1995 the preliminary certificates will be replaced with an updated range of modules.

BEBOH also offers higher level examinations (the Certificate and Diploma) for specialist occupational hygienists. The Certificate denotes all round competence in the technical aspects of occupational hygiene, whilst the Diploma is the professional qualification for senior hygienists and hygiene managers.

A Lead Body for occupational safety and health has been formed by the government and it is currently introducing National Vocational Qualifications. These are intended to test practical competence in health and safety skills such as risk assessment. The qualifications are still at the pilot stage and are not yet established.

Technical competency may be all that is required for some low level jobs in occupational hygiene. For most hygienists, though, it is no longer sufficient for the hygienist just to have technical skills. Effective performance depends on an ability to get results as much as on technical knowledge. This may involve:

- influencing employees to use the control measures provided properly;
- monitoring and controlling other hygiene staff to perform optimally;
- influencing managers to make or support decisions.

Getting results in this way, through people, is the science of management. It requires attitudes, knowledge and skills which traditionally have not been taught to hygienists.

A hygienist with technical but not management ability functions as a specialist, called on only when required to supply data for others to make decisions. In contrast, the occupational hygiene manager has a major influence on company policies, direction and performance. Management ability is therefore a core requirement for all senior hygienists and consultants. Key skills which must be mastered include:

- communication (both written and oral)
- decision making
- problem solving
- negotiating
- planning
- time management
- project management
- risk management
- counselling and disciplining
- training and development
- motivation and leadership
- performance monitoring
- auditing
- quality assurance
- budgetary control.

Consultants may need additional tuition in areas such as sales and marketing techniques.

These management skills cannot operate in a vacuum: they must be used against a background of the organization's culture, procedures, current status and plans. In particular, the hygienist should be thoroughly conversant with:

- the nature of the business (the products or services offered, their relative importance and prospects)
- the organizational structure
- management style, systems and procedures
- manufacturing methods
- the roles of trade unions and safety representatives
- the financial performance of the company and the occupational hygiene department/function.

To be effective, the hygienist must see him or herself as an integral part of the organization with an interest in its overall performance. This is true even of an external consultant.

ACCREDITATION OF HYGIENISTS

It is sometimes assumed that a high level manager of health, safety and environment does not need detailed technical knowledge of the subject since he or she is concerned only with policy and management issues. This is a dangerous course. So many decisions in occupational hygiene depend on a proper interpretation of complex data and observations. Likewise it is unsafe to assume that because samples were taken by a competent technician that a production manager will be able to make the right decisions from the results.

At present anyone can call him or herself an occupational hygienist, and many people do so without having any proper qualifications in the subject. This has caused problems particularly in the fields of asbestos abatement and more recently COSHH assessments, where commercial consultancies have proliferated. Unqualified consultants have left dissatisfied clients, earned bad press for the profession and put employees' health at risk.

At the same time, cultural changes are affecting the way occupational hygiene is practised. Hitherto professionalism has been informal. It was derived from the expertise of the individuals, not from rules or regulations governing their conduct. But the status of professionals in society is changing. Their authority is more open to question and they must be seen to justify their arguments and status as never before (Watkins, Drury and Preddy, 1992).

This has led to changes in the profession. For instance, the Institute of Occupational Hygienists now proposes to introduce a formal scheme of continuing professional development (IOH, 1994) to ensure that professionals stay up to date. The Institute is also reviewing its Code of Ethics to ensure that the public is adequately protected. The nature of the hygienist's role means that ethical questions will inevitably arise. For instance:

- the confidentiality of personal occupational health data must be protected;
- potential conflicts can arise between the loyalties of hygienists to employers, workers, clients and the law;
- employers may (deliberately or unintentionally) impose constraints on the freedom of the hygienist to carry out his or her duties, e.g. access to sites, equipment available, time allowed, level of supporting staff;
- the use of junior staff for fieldwork raises questions about the adequacy of supervision;
- advertising and sales practices of consultancies may need to be subject to ethical constraints.

Of course, the public has no protection unless the hygienist is a qualified professional. This has persuaded many hygienists to seek some kind of legal recognition. It may take the form of title recognition, whereby only qualified occupational hygienists are allowed to use the name, or it may involve licensing.

Pressure for legal recognition has been highest in the USA, where asbestos and lead abatement practices have aroused public attention. California and Tennessee now have legislation on recognition and Illinois has a licensing law. In Europe, The Netherlands has become the first country where qualified hygienists have to be on a government register. For the rest of the EU it is still a case of let the buyer beware.

These points also raise deeper questions. Should the provision of occupational hygiene services by regulated? Should they be provided by the state as in Eastern European countries? Is it socially and politically practicable to do either or should the market economy decide? It may be that a balanced blend of different types of services provides the optimal conditions for the protection of health, but how can this balance be achieved? How can it be assured that every employee and every company has access to occupational hygiene expertise when needed? Or will we instead see a simplistic and inefficient approach based on compliance with OELs?

REFERENCES

ACGIH (1993) *1993–1994 Threshold Limit Values for Chemical Substances and Physical Agents and Biological Exposure Indices,* American Conference of Governmental Industrial Hygienists, Cincinnati, OH, USA.

Allen, J. (1983) The development of a full-shift, true breathing zone personal air sampler and its application to lead workers. University of Manchester PhD Thesis.

Allen, J., Bellinger E.G. and Higgins R.I. (1981) A full shift true breathing zone sampler and its application to lead workers. *Proceedings of the Institution of Mechanical Engineers*, **195**(25), 325–8.

Bailey, S.R. and Miles, D.P. (1984) A practical method of improving the efficiency and value of air sampling, in *Papers Presented to the Institute in 1983*, Report No. 4, Institute of Occupational Hygienists, Derby, UK.

Bloor, W.A., Eardley, R.E. and Dinsdale, A. (1968) A gravimetric personal dust sampler. *Annals of Occupational Hygiene*, **11**(1), 81–6.

Deacon, A. (1994) The role of safety in Total Quality Management. *The Safety and Health Practitioner*, **12**(1), 18–21.

Dewell, P. (1989) *Some Applications of Statistics in Occupational Hygiene*, H & H Scientific Consultants, Leeds, UK.

Greeno, J.L., Hedstrom, G.S. and Diberto, M. (1988) *The Environmental, Health and Safety Auditor's Handbook*, Arthur D. Little, Cambridge, Massachusetts, USA.

Handy, C.B. (1985) *Understanding Organizations*, Penguin Group, London.

Health and Safety Commission (1992) *Annual Report 1991/92*, HSE Books, Sudbury, UK.

Higgins, R.I. (1982) The statistical basis of survey and routine occupational hygiene sampling, in *Sampling,Statistics and Epidemiology*, Report No. 2, Institute of Occupational Hygienists, Derby, UK.

HSE (1993) *EH64 Occupational Exposure Limits: Criteria Document Summaries* (1993 edn and supplement), HSE Books, Sudbury, UK.

HSE (1994) *EH40/94 Occupational Exposure Limits 1994*, HSE Books, Sudbury, UK.

IOH (1993) *Membership Information Pack*, Institute of Occupational Hygienists, Derby, UK.

IOH (1994) *Continuing Professional Development in IOH*. Consultation Paper: Institute of Occupational Hygienists, Derby, UK.

King, E. (1980) Techniques for the measurement of cadmium in air, in *Occupational Exposure to Cadmium*, Report on Seminar, Cadmium Development Association, London, pp. 7–11.

Kromhout, H., Symanski, E. and Rappaport, S.M. (1993) A comprehensive evaluation of within and between-worker components of occupational exposure to chemical agents. *Annals of Occupational Hygiene*, **37**(3), 253–70.

Mole, J. (1993) *Mind your Manners*, Nicholas Brealey, London.

Ogden T.L. *et al.* (1993) Dust from cotton manufacture: changing from static to personal sampling. *Annals of Occupational Hygiene*, **37**(3), 271–85.

OHR (1994) *Occupational Health Review*, March–April, 24–7.

Ramazzini, B. (1940) *De Morbis Artificum*, 2nd edn (trans. W.C. Wright), Chicago University Press, Chicago.

Rappaport S.M. (1991) Assessment of long term exposures to toxic substances in air. *Annals of Occupational Hygiene*, **35**(1), 61–122.

Robens, Lord (1972) Safety and Health at Work: Report of the Committee 1970–72, HMSO, London.

Watkins, J. Drury, L. and Preddy, N. (1992) *From Evolution to Revolution: the Pressures on Professional Life in the Nineties*, University of Bristol, UK.

Workwell Program, Workers' Compensation Board, Toronto, Ontario, Canada.

First aid and paramedics

9

Matthew C. Cullen

INTRODUCTION

First aid at work provision is subject to three different government regulations in the United Kingdom. This chapter gives a broad outline of some of the main elements of these regulations. It sets out to widen the reader's perspectives, and to highlight some of the deficiencies and pitfalls in the whole field of first aid at work generally; and whilst not expecting to cover every possible future development, some indication is given of the paths which these might take.

The earliest legislation which required employers to make first aid provision for employees was that enshrined in an Order in 1917 (Statutory Instrument and Order No. 1067, 1917). Since that Order, successive pieces of legislation have added to – or strengthened – the legal requirements. In 1961 (Factories Act 1961), the first major changes for many years were made. Amongst these was the provision of very broad guidelines for the content of first aid boxes in different industries and the naming of seven bodies to train first aiders to work in factories. Similar changes affecting commercial premises and others followed two years later (Offices, Shops and Railways Premises Act 1963). In neither piece of legislation was any advice given on the content of courses, examination procedure or qualification of those concerned with training or examining.

Until the 1970s, all first aid matters were controlled by the Factory Inspectorate's Medical Inspectors. Following the establishment of the Employment Medical Advisory Service (EMAS) in 1972 (Employment Medical Advisory Service Act 1972), all responsibility for health, including first aid, was passed from the Medical Inspectors. EMAS (which became part of the Health and Safety Executive (HSE) in 1974) appointed both Employment Nursing Advisors (ENAs) and Employment Medical Advisors (EMAs) and part of their respective duties was to collate information on the standard of first aid practice and services in all places of work including, for example, factories, shops, offices, hospitals, educational establishments and laboratories. Their findings resulted in a decision to replace the existing outdated legislation with completely new regulations. Thus, the Health and Safety (First Aid) Regulations 1981 were enacted giving HSE powers to deal with all aspects of first aid training and provision in every workplace.

FIRST AID 1994

HSE, the regulatory body in England, Scotland and Wales (Northern Ireland has separate arrangements), is responsible for enforcing the regulations governing the provision of first aid at work. The Health and Safety (First Aid) Regulations 1981, Offshore Installations and Pipelines Works (First Aid) Regulations 1989 and the Diving Operations at Work Regulations 1990 between them cover every type of work and give the interpretation of all these regulations. Information on who can provide training for first aiders, numbers required in workplace, content of first aid boxes, syllabus and examination procedures is contained in guidance and Approved Codes of Practice to the regulations. Arrangements for refresher courses are also covered.

Some employers are still confused about the type of training a first aider needs and commonly believe that any type of first aid certificate will suffice. The HSE is very firm in this respect stating unequivocally that training in public (i.e. general) first aid is unsuitable for any type of workplace because the type of conditions encountered therein can be of a particular nature depending on the kind of industry. Therefore it is important that first aiders in workplaces are trained in first aid relevant to work. Because of this stipulation those trained solely to attend public events to care for the general public would not be acceptable.

Any organization which sets out to train first aiders in accordance with the Health and Safety (First Aid) Regulations 1981 (HSFAR) must satisfy HSE on a number of details before approval for that organization is considered. The proposed syllabus must accord with that contained in the Approved Code of Practice. Any topic not directly work related may only be taught after the course has been completed. The whole course must be directed to the types of incident which can be encountered at work. Emphasis must be given to specific injuries (chemical burns is a prime example) which would not normally be found in a public first aid course. This requirement has caused some difficulty in the past for the large voluntary training bodies – St John Ambulance, St Andrew's Ambulance and the British Red Cross Society – because they provided most of the first aid cover at public events and carried out most of the first aid at work training in England, Scotland and Wales. The regulations meant that they had to provide different types of training.

The voluntary aid organizations are not the sole providers of first aid at work training courses. Many other organizations, numbering some 1400 by spring 1994 (and this number is increasing), are approved by HSE. Included in these are some large companies which, for financial saving coupled with the need to have training related directly to their own type of operation, are also approved. The regulations covering the offshore and diving industries also provide for the training of first aiders. Since the nature of these latter undertakings is more hazardous, the training is different in syllabus to that contained in the HSFAR. Training courses are longer and offshore first aiders have access to more equipment. Because the trainers and examiners must have worked in either the offshore or diving industries, and also due to the smaller numbers of people employed, the number of organizations providing training is smaller, and by spring 1994 between 20 and 30 had gained approval.

The issue of experience required amongst trainers and examiners is another area which many do not fully understand or appreciate. HSE require that those who are to either train or examine must themselves have had experience as first aiders at work or have been concerned with first aid services in a professional capacity. Both nurses and doctors employed in industry/commerce are covered by this requirement. A nurse who works in a hospital accident and emergency department, or in general wards, will not have the necessary understanding of working conditions outside that environment to enable him/her to teach or examine adequately those who will provide care in industrial or commercial settings. Although there is no specific requirement for occupational health nurses to undertake a trainers' course – which all lay trainers must attend – many do so to learn the basics of teaching. Sadly, for whatever reason, not all occupational health physicians see the need to equip themselves in the same way. Many doctors who, prior to the introduction of the HSFAR, taught and examined first aiders had never visited a factory or attended a first aid course as a participant. It must be self-evident that if health professionals are to enter the field of training and/or examining they should, at the very least, have attended a course themselves. Without this knowledge it will prove difficult for them to be fully involved with courses. Where examiners are concerned there are great differences between styles and interpretation and all those who proffer themselves in this role must be trained in the art and technique of examining, yet this important issue has received little attention from those approved to train first aiders.

There are a great many conditions that organizations that wish to provide first aid at work training must satisfy before HSE will give them approval. Some of these have already been described and it may help the reader to learn of some of the others. Details outlining methods of teaching, equipment to be used, samples of lesson material, and the size and type of premises must be provided. Trainers are not permitted to examine those whom they have trained and examination accommodation must be described. Privacy for students during the individual practical examination must be assured. HSE's ENAs and EMAs monitor courses and examinations to ensure that all conditions are being met. Where deficiencies are encountered, these are discussed at the time with the individual concerned. The coordinator for the course is notified by letter so that the fault can be rectified. If it is not, or there is blatant disregard of any important condition, then HSE may remove the approval for that organization to continue to provide training (and in a small number of cases it has already taken this step). There is an appeals procedure for any organization to follow if it feels that it has been unfairly treated.

The numbers of ENAs and EMAs employed by EMAS are relatively small and monitoring first aid courses and examinations is part of their duties, yet this aspect does not have the high profile which is probably necessary in view of the large number of approved courses being held each year. Other methods of ensuring compliance with regulations need to be examined and one of these is self-monitoring although it may not be without drawbacks. Cross-monitoring between approved organizations is also a possibility. An independent body appointed by HSE to oversee monitoring but without any powers to act would seem at least worthy of consideration. HSE, as the regulating authority, would be able to take appropriate action in cases where adverse reports on the standards being achieved by an approved organization were presented.

Although all these details may appear to be unnecessarily restrictive, HSE is committed to ensuring that training achieves the highest possible standard. The use of strict guidance and other measures will ultimately ensure that the first aider is trained to a reasonably high national standard and is thus able to deliver the best possible care to those who rely upon his or her expertise whilst pursuing their daily tasks.

Within the scope of HSFAR is the training for those first aiders who work in industries where special hazards exist. These are termed 'Specific Hazards', and cover the use of cyanide and hydrofluoric acid because these chemicals can be treated with special antidotes. In addition, the Factories Act 1961 section 30 requires employees to be trained in the use of medical oxygen when it is to be used solely for the purpose of rescue of employees from airless conditions. Training courses for these three special circumstances are provided by approved bodies. Whilst the treatment involved with the use of cyanide and hydrofluoric acid is easily understood, there is often confusion regarding treatment with oxygen. HSE does not approve of the general use of oxygen by first aiders at work for purely medical conditions – respiratory disease is an example – because of the problems of diagnosis involved as well as for other reasons. It is not essential for those employees trained to deal with the above conditions to hold a full first aid at work certificate. Very often once an employee has attended a specific hazards course, he or she feels that further training would be of benefit and can pursue the matter with his or her employer.

Apart from the legislative aspect of first aid in the workplace there is a more down-to-earth side for consideration. It is often said – with a great deal of truth – that once employers have appointed the necessary personnel to provide a first aid service they then give them no more thought. Whilst employers pay for the costs of courses, they tend to forget that the first aider(s) were originally employed for an entirely different purpose and it is rare for first aiders to be employed solely for the purpose of administering first aid. Due recompense for undertaking a second task – providing first aid care – is not always made although some employers do make small payments, usually on an annual basis. These men and women are the sole providers of first aid treatment for employees who suffer injury or become ill at work and employers do not seem to realize the heavy burden of responsibility that first aiders carry, because if they did so they would certainly recognize the need for reward. Reward can be made in a number of ways apart from cash payments; extra holidays, or goods (which may attract income tax penalties) may be used, for example. First aiders then have tangible evidence that their efforts are appreciated.

FIRST AIDERS – THE LEGAL POSITION

First aiders and employers worry about their legal responsibilities in delivering first aid to fellow workers. There has been little case law over the years to give direction in every circumstance. Provided that the first aiders do not attempt any treatment, or give advice, outside the parameters of their training and also that what they do or say is acceptable in the eyes of experts, there should be no need to worry. The HSE has provided a useful definition of correct first aid practice as (personal communication):

> ... when first aiders act in accordance with the standards of the ordinary skilled first aider exercising and professing to have that

special skill of a first aider. What will amount to the ordinary standard is a question of law to be decided by the courts. However, where it can be shown that the first aider acted in accordance with general and approved practice current at the time in question, then he is unlikely to be viewed as having fallen short of the skill required of him. Even if there is no complete agreement as to what is approved practice approved by a responsible body of medical opinion, this will be sufficient.

How is a court to assess what is 'approved practice'? Clearly it would have to receive evidence in some form of medical opinion on the relevant matter. A court will inevitably derive considerable assistance in assessing first aid practice by reference to [an authoritative first aid] manual; this will not be conclusive with regard to any issue arising from the application of first aid in a particular case, since it has been accepted by the courts that with regard to matters of diagnosis and treatment genuine differences of opinion arise.

FIRST AID – LIFTING THE VEIL

Much has been made nationally in the United Kingdom of the benefits of European Union (EU) membership. In most spheres of commerce, industry and healthcare activities allowances have been made for the influence and impact of EU involvement. First aid at work is one area that has been totally neglected for discussion on common standards of first aid across the EU. Recently the United Kingdom Resuscitation Council has joined with the European Resuscitation Council to help establish mutually agreed standards of care and treatment in resuscitation measures. There exists a growing need for full cooperation between EU member states and Scandinavian countries so that dialogue can commence to establish policy and standards for first aid. One of the advantages of common standards would be a material contribution to raising the treatment levels across the European Union and Scandinavia. As a first move, new legislation will need to define the term 'first aid' for purely legal reasons. At present, this is used loosely to cover both injury and illness. The First Aid at Work – Approved Code of Practice 1990 defines first aid as '. . . in cases where a person will need help from a medical practitioner or nurse, treatment for the purposes of preserving life and minimising the consequences of injury and illness until such help is obtained'. However the Oxford Dictionary defines first aid as 'treatment given to an injured person before a doctor comes', and Blacks Medical Dictionary refers to first aid entirely in terms of injury. In both cases, the inclusion of illness under the term of first aid is omitted. This suggests that a more appropriate term might be emergency aid in all future legislation because the term can have a broader meaning. Many countries have already established varying levels of first aid provision at work. EU legislation would need to cover a basic standard for all workplaces. It should set standards for the establishment of panels of trainers and examiners, who themselves have been suitably trained for these roles. Guidance will be needed to provide a basic syllabus content and examination procedure and to decide on the period between, and nature of, refresher courses. A very necessary concomitant would be dedicated, multi-lingual first aid manuals. In the United Kingdom there is a plethora of first aid manuals most of which would be for general – as opposed to first aid at work – use. The St John Ambulance organization has, in the light of recent research findings (Cullen, 1992), taken the necessary steps to produce a manual (St John Ambulance Supplies) solely for the first aid at work course students. Some other organizations, usually large companies that are approved to train their own personnel, have also prepared their own internal manuals. However, most first aiders use a first aid manual which contains information and treatments wholly in-appropriate for work situations. Lastly, another necessary area will need commonly agreed standards and that is health of would-be first aiders. A 64-year-old first aider with a chronic chest condition will be unlikely to be able to resuscitate an employee if the first aider has had first to run up a flight of stairs. Currently, there is little restriction beyond that exercised by responsible first aid training organizations. Restrictions relating to fitness and general health would need to be examined in some depth.

SYLLABUS CONTENT

The present syllabus used in the teaching of first aid is exceptionally detailed for first aid at work. There are topics included which take up unnecessarily large amounts of teaching time and two of these readily spring to mind. Most training bodies spend an average of four hours on fractures yet the vast majority of first aiders are unlikely to have to deal with a fracture at work. The National Health Service Emergency Ambulance Service has a current response time of approximately 12 minutes in urban areas (obviously this time will vary in different parts of the country) and by the time the first aider has carried out suppor-tive treatment the Emergency Ambulance with highly trained and experienced paramedics will have arrived. These personnel are far more skilled than the average first aider in transporting an employee with a fracture. There should be no need for the first aider to move the injured person beyond keeping him or her out of danger. The inclusion of fractures and their treatment in the syllabus should be reviewed or direction given to training bodies on reducing of time spent on these topics. Transportation of casualties is another topic in the syllabus which, for the same reasons, would benefit from review. (However, these remarks apply equally to the syllabus for public first aid.) As far as the whole syllabus is concerned, a totally new approach could be profitably considered. Industry falls broadly into several categories – engineering, chemicals and construction are the main ones. A syllabus encompassing principles of first aid, resuscitation, and very basic anatomy and physiology, based on what first aiders do – rather than based on a belief of what they need to know – would form the main core, after which the first aider would attend modules with training directed to particular types of injury encountered in his or her work-place. A final module would deal with medical emergencies and their management. This type of training readily permits the use of continuous assessment rather then the stereotyped theoretical examination currently used.

Presently, most training is carried out over a four-day period, with a contact period of six hours daily. This system appeals to employers because the first aider is able to complete the course within a week. However, training over four consecutive days is taxing in the extreme. The first aider has to absorb a great deal of material. Due allowance cannot be made for those who are slow learners, have difficulty in writing their own notes, or who experience other difficulties associated with an intensive course. Because of all these factors, future training must look at an entirely new approach. Most training uses the positive approach, i.e. how to proceed when injury or illness occurs at work. There are some occasions when it is more profitable to tell the first aider what not to do, yet this approach in training is rarely used. At times doing too much can be as bad as doing too little. Perhaps extending the course to a day a week for four weeks, or one half day a week for eight weeks would be a gentler approach. These possible systems are not perfect and could affect employees who are shift workers, and would inevitably have administrative consequences for employers.

FIRST AID EXAMINATIONS

How first aiders are examined to probe the depth of their learning and knowledge is a topic which exercises many minds. Generally speaking, the current practice is to administer a theoretical test – which may be written, or a multiple-choice questionnaire, and a practical test. The latter is the most important one, since it will demonstrate the first aider's ability to perform resuscitative techniques adequately. Whatever the answer, the use of four-day courses may tend to suggest that the first aider is being prepared to pass an examination rather than for the practice of first aid over the years ahead.

NEW TECHNOLOGY IN FIRST AID

Slowly, first aid training organizations are beginning to use some of the new technologies. Possibly the first ventures in these fields have been the use of videotape programmes used by the St John Ambulance and British Red Cross Society. Another first was the computer interactive 'Save A Life' program devised by Dr Burridge (Burridge, 1986). This program was designed to run on the BBC computers and, as the title implies, deals with resuscitation. Some large industrial undertakings have also produced videotape training sets for use inhouse. The advantages of using in-house programmes are many, perhaps the greatest being that they can cover exactly the situation that the trainer wants so that particular points of treatment can be emphasized.

The general approach to training is still didactic directed amongst training bodies. With the exception of the quoted examples, little effort appears to have been made to explore the use of interactive video programmes. Computer-assisted learning with all the benefits this could bring for refresher courses has still not been exploited. Distance learning schemes are a method which has proved itself in other fields and the use of this method in first aid training is in its infancy. However, the method requires – in terms of first aid training – the experience and facilities of a major professional educational body to test its use in this field. Universities and equivalent institutions are well placed to design and tutor courses, which require a great deal of commitment in terms of time, finance and expertise if they are to succeed. It is doubtful whether any major first aid training body can provide all the essential elements to run a distance learning scheme at the present time, although the subject is debatable. All training course material could not be covered by these techniques, since the necessity for practical training still remains, but a sizeable part of the syllabus now in use could be converted to this type of training. Despite high developmental costs the system has many great advantages. First aiders can learn at their own pace, they can revise at any time – even between courses – and the time spent away from work could be reduced. This could help particularly small firms that find it difficult to release employees for the four consecutive day course because of work commitments. A flexible approach should allow for educational and treatment changes easily and frequently.

In occupational health and other fields training in many areas is becoming competency based. Whilst there may be a case for using competency as an assessment tool in first aid at work training, the final decision to use competency-based systems must rest on whether or not it will materially improve the delivery of first aid. A pilot study would soon easily prove or disprove the value of competency assessment in first aid at work training.

RESEARCH

Over the last 77 years of the practice of first aid at work, little attempt to research the practice of first aid and its teaching has been made. It is only in the last nine years that any research in these areas has been undertaken and published. The first of these, in 1986, dealt with cardio-pulmonary resuscitation (Glendon et al., 1986) and examined skill decay amongst first aiders in relation to their ability to perform resuscitation properly after a fixed period. The second study was concerned with the wider aspects of retention of learned material excluding resuscitation (Cullen, 1992) after training. A third study has dealt with devices for use when performing mouth-to-mouth resuscitation (Howie et al., 1992). The first two of these studies are areas of major concern for first aid training bodies and clearly demonstrate a need for urgent further and deeper research. In recent years the major voluntary training bodies have provided most of the first aid at work training and consequently must have received a high income from this source. But none of them, with the exception of a questionnaire-type study by St John Ambulance into injuries amongst school children, apparently has seen any need or felt duty-bound to devote any of this income towards furthering research. This lack of interest must raise questions about their total interests in providing training. If the delivery and practice of first aid is to achieve high standards, then many of its aspects need research. Training bodies must examine their whole approach to training methods, treatment practices and beliefs, and equipment because these are now topics for action and concern. Work is necessary to probe both the attitude of employers and the methods they use to choose employees to act as first aiders, and also the attitude of fellow employees to first aiders. Another area which will benefit from research is the content and frequency of refresher courses, although this may be for the regulatory body, rather than the training organizations, to pursue. The need for first aiders to self-refresh is paramount if they are to keep their knowledge current. Generally speaking, first aiders will readily admit that they seldom refer to their first aid manuals after they have completed training. Few employers are aware of or recognize this need. A study to examine the extent to which first aiders and their employers set aside time for revision would be of value in helping to determine the optimum period between refresher courses.

ETHNIC FIRST AIDERS

In some areas with large communities of minority ethnic groups, English has become the second language in many workplaces, with employees communicating entirely, whilst at work, in their mother tongues. To satisfy legal requirements and the ethnic workforce's needs, many employers displayed safety and other signs in appropriate languages. Not a great deal has been done by HSE approved first aid training bodies to foresee that special arrangements are needed to deal with the problem surrounding training for Asians, Europeans and Chinese first aiders. In a few instances, courses are being offered in Chinese (British Red Cross, Manchester presently run this type of course). There also exists the possibility that special approaches or procedures may be needed to satisfy the religious and other beliefs of some ethnic groups. These considerations must be examined by those who are concerned with first aid issues, whether the interest be in training, regulation or administration of first aid to employees.

PARAMEDICS IN THE UNITED KINGDOM

With the possible exception of the armed services, paramedic activity in the United Kingdom slowly developed with the employment of offshore rig and diver medics in the 1960s. Undoubtedly the first medics so employed were ex-servicemen (female medics were not employed until the 1980s) who probably came from the Royal Navy or Special Services. These were medics specially trained by the Armed Forces Medical Training School and were used to working in remote and unusual conditions with little medical support and therefore were uniquely qualified to work in the dangerous environment offshore. However, not all employers in those early days sought experienced medics and there were many pitfalls waiting for those medics who did not always provide a high level of care through lack of training and experience. Within the author's experience there was at least one employer in the offshore field who advertised for newly qualified nurses in the early 1970s. These nurses, with little or no post-basic experience, were expected by the employer to work in a hostile, hazardous and isolated environment with no on-site medical supervision or other professional help. Despite this, the vast majority of medics did provide a very good service. The medics soon recognized the need for further and continuing training and the Offshore Medical Club was formed with the guidance of Dr J. Mann in Aberdeen in the early 1970s.

This club provided a common meeting ground and an early successful opportunity to provide continuing education in the form of informal talks and lectures. The Employment Medical Advisory Service in the mid-1970s started to collate information on the need for training for rig medics on a more formal basis. Once gathered and interpreted the necessity for discussion with employers and others concerned as well as with other government departments became evident. Consequent to prolonged consultations the need for regulation to cover all aspects of offshore care became very obvious. As a result and after a consultation document had been issued, the Offshore Installations and Pipelines Works (First Aid) Regulations 1989 were enacted under the aegis of the HSE. These regulations and accompanying Code of Practice set out for employers and all those concerned with the training of rig medics and the delivery of care offshore, details of training courses and examinations for both rig medics and offshore first aiders, and of suitable treatment accommodation and equipment. The bigger employers in the industry had foreseen the need to train and support their rig medics and offshore first aiders, although smaller employers still paid scant attention to providing similar support. The regulations, at least and at last, ensured that a highly efficient level of care for employees offshore was established. Hot on the heels of this legislation, HSE introduced new legislation – the Diving Operations at Work Regulations (Amended) 1990 for diver medics and first aiders.

In the meantime, between 1972 and 1974, the Brighton Ambulance Service began a local training scheme for Ambulance Service personnel. This was ultimately to lead to a nationally agreed training scheme for ambulance paramedics. In Cornwall in 1988 the first Air Ambulance Service using paramedics was set up on a voluntary basis. The last development for Ambulance Service paramedics was the use of rapid response motor-cycle mounted paramedics in some of the larger cities within the last two years. Today the vast majority of paramedics are employed by the National Health Service. The training scheme for all Ambulance Service paramedics is intense and thorough.

The syllabus used is the same throughout the country, possibly with some minor changes from area to area. Because it is nationally agreed it surpasses the early US system in which there is a national core system and each state adds on modules to its own requirements. This system has many drawbacks not the least being that a paramedic who wishes to move from one state to another probably has to undergo further training for the new post.

At present, all paramedics in the various fields of armed services, offshore and diving and the Ambulance Service are highly trained. Since their appearance in the field of emergency care has been comparatively recent in terms of first aid at work, there are very few, if

202 First aid and paramedics

any, solely employed as paramedics in industry. It is unlikely that this will change much in the foreseeable future, yet the possibility remains that in the event of redundancies in their fields of work, some paramedics may seek posts in various types of industry. Whether they would be acceptable legally as first aiders without formal training under the Health and Safety (First Aid) Regulations 1981 is a matter for the HSE to decide. Again from the purely legal side, professional opinion as to whether they could practise their full paramedic skills in an emergency would be necessary.

Paramedics will still have a place in their respective places of work but it is improbable that wider opportunities for them will open up in industry in the existing climate. With the passage of time there may be developments in some industries for paramedics with their special skills to be employed – that time is some distance in the future.

In mid-1994 the HSE began advocating competency-based training. The current Regulations Approved Code of Practice and Guidance Notes have been reviewed and a Consultative Document was issued in the autumn of 1994.

REFERENCES

Burridge, P. (1986) Save-A-Life Disk Interactive Program, Birch Hill Hospital, Rochdale, Greater Manchester, UK.

Cullen, M.C. (1992) First Aid retention of knowledge survey. *Health and Safety Executive Research Paper No. 32*, HSE Books, Sudbury, UK.

Employment Medical Advisory Service Act 1972. HMSO, London.

Factories Act 1961. HMSO, London.

Glendon, A.I., Blaylock, S.S., McKenna, S.P. and Hunt, K. (1986) Cardio-pulmonary resuscitation skill decay: Current Research Findings. *British Health and Safety Society Newsletter*, 13, 14–18.

Howie, R.M., Hagen, S., McLaren, W. and Sinclair, K.W. (1992) Development of test methods for evaluating the effectiveness of manual resuscitation devices. *Institute of Occupational Medicine Report*, TM/92/09, Edinburgh, Scotland.

Offices, Shops and Railway Premises Act 1963. HMSO, London.

St John Ambulance Supplies *St John Ambulance First Aid at Work Manual* (Foundation Course). St John Ambulance Supplies, London.

Statutory Instrument and Order No. 1067, 1917. Order in regard to Ambulance and first aid Arrangements at Blast Furnaces, Copper Mills, Foundries and Metal Works. HMSO, London.

PART THREE

Research in occupational health 10

Indira Ashton and
Ian Wright

INTRODUCTION

It is a well-known fact that work can cause or exacerbate disease. Data collected as part of the 1990 Labour Force Survey (Hodgson *et al.*, 1993) revealed the degree of work related ill health in particular occupations. Though the data is based upon individuals' own perceptions of their health and its connection with their work, it gave an insight into aspects of occupational ill health for which there is little evidence elsewhere.

One of the most commonly reported work related illnesses for both manual and non-manual occupations was musculo-skeletal conditions. These included upper limb disorders caused by work; associated with these were tenosynovitis, carpal tunnel syndrome and tennis elbow and some respondents felt that the cause was repetitive strain injury. For manual occupations, the commonly reported illnesses were the long-term consequences of trauma and poisoning, disease of the lungs and deafness. For non-manual occupations, other leading causes were stress, depression and, for office-based occupations, headache and eye strain.

The survey identified 20 categories of self-report work related illness, for each of 18 occupational groups. Work in mining, construction and metal, electrical and other processing sectors, transport and materials moving, farming, fishing, forestry and nursing displayed higher than average overall risks. Certain occupations showed a higher than average risk of a particular illness. Examples include stress and depression caused by work was four times greater in teachers than the average for other occupations; risk of back problems in nurses was three times the average; and risk of headache and eye strain in clerical workers was twice the average for other occupations.

Musculo-skeletal conditions also gave rise to most lost time from work, followed by stress or depression and the late consequences of trauma and poisoning. The latter two were also the most commonly reported as causing the individual to change jobs.

So, does recent research in occupational health address these issues?

Schilling (1993) feels that promoting occupational health in its broadest sense still depends on clinical skills to assess fitness for work and to identify responses to adverse factors in the environment. Opportunities for research are extensive and include identifying the extent and severity of injury or illness due to adverse environmental agents and other factors, assessing fitness among the disabled and enabling them to be gainfully employed, improving techniques for measuring work exposures and human responses to adverse work factors, and evaluating intervention procedures.

Occupational health research in the United Kingdom has been diagnosed by Harrington (1990) as a 'rather sickly patient'. He advances the view that most published work concerns the investigation of work effects on health or health effects on work, with insufficient attention being paid to research into the prevention of occupational health hazards and the delivery of occupational health services. Coggon (1990) continued this theme, suggesting that there is an imbalance between the research actually being done in the United Kingdom and what practising occupational physicians feel they need. He cites evidence given at a meeting of the Society of Occupational Medicine (SOM) Research and Development Panel, where a review of the two British specialist occupational medicine journals (*British Journal of Industrial Medicine*, now known as *Occupational and Environmental Medicine*, and *Journal of the Society of Occupational Medicine*, now known as *Occupational Medicine*) revealed a strong emphasis on papers elucidating hazards in the workplace. This was contrasted with the response of SOM members to a questionnaire, which had indicated that their interest lay mainly in the effective management of established hazards and the problems of selection and placement of employees.

This state of affairs is of concern to occupational health professionals, who care about the future of the speciality. There have been a number of initiatives by both the SOM and the Faculty of Occupational Medicine of the Royal College of Physicians to remedy the situation. In an ideal world, there would be a controlling body directing, regulating and funding a systematic occupational health research programme focusing on specific needs. This is unlikely to occur, but hopefully, having recognized the problems, occupational health professionals will, by self-regulation, direct their research efforts to fields which will meet needs and answer specific questions. This should move the profession away from the 'must be a good idea' school of occupational health practice (Slovak, 1993) towards practice based on sound scientific research.

The costs of good quality research into occupational health are substantial as it often involves multidisciplinary investigatory teams of physicians, occupational hygienists, occupational health nurses, statisticians or epidemiologists, bioengineers, computer specialists and others working together. Added to this is the multiyear project duration, participation by specific industry employers and employees and the inevitable travel expenses. The data collected must be relevant to the quantification of human health risks in association with well characterized exposures. It is now more cost effective to design studies of human populations which compare reliable exposure information with evidence of disease in the exposed population and to establish safe levels of exposure. Disease related to exposure should be assessed at the margin of detectability with traditional epidemiological tools. In more recent times, biomarkers have been developed that are minimally invasive, or non-invasive, to detect and quantify exposure, identify susceptibility to an untoward response and uncover the early indication of disease process. It therefore appears that there is adequate justification for the continued investigation of occupational disease through studies of exposed populations.

Length of studies requires comment. A study collecting longitudinal data over a five-year period will actually take eight or more years to perform, from design to completion of analyses and interpretation and publication of results.

Some attempts have been made to identify the problems requiring future research in specific occupational groups, for example Diamond (1990) identified the research needs of the transport industry. These included the clinical assessment of applicants for safety critical jobs, such as drivers, the design of jobs in both ergonomic and psychological aspects, and the effects on health of components of exhaust gas emissions. Baxter (1991) and Heap (1993) addressed the needs of the health care professions. They identified the increasing use of technology and greater recognition of psychological problems, together with the risks of infection, as areas requiring research. The health effects of specific hazards such as gluteraldehyde and cytotoxic agents, as well as the effects of physical problems such as back pain, and the psychological stress of long hours and being part of a caring profession were also identified. McKiernan (1990), writing about the occupational health research needs of the engineering industry, cited the problems of rapidly changing technology in an intensely competitive environment. He identified the problem of providing a flexible occupational health service, able to keep pace with the industry while remaining accessible and responsive to employees by providing a relevant and effective occupational health service.

A review of the published occupational health research work emanating from British centres in the last few years gives an insight into those areas of current interest to researchers and indicates whether these research projects are dealing with the real needs of the occupational health profession. More details about some of the research papers are given below, grouped roughly into body system or area of concern and arranged in alphabetical order of grouping.

ACCIDENTS

In the UK, national statistics on accidents that occur at work depend upon the information acquired through the Reporting of Injuries, Diseases and Dangerous Occurrences Regulations 1985 which came into effect in 1986. It places an obligation on the employer to report to the Health and Safety Executive accidents and incidents in various categories and the ones in which a three-day absence occurs. According to Harker et al. (1991) figures on fatal accidents tend to be well documented, but data on major injuries not resulting in death tend to be under-reported and such a system means that less severe injuries, leading to fewer than three days' incapacity to work, go unreported. Such minor injuries may impose a burden on both employer and the accident and emergency services of the National Health Service and represent an area where preventive action could prove cost effective.

Harker et al. (1991) undertook a prospective survey of patients attending the Central Accident and Emergency Department and Eye Casualty Department in Aberdeen to determine the contribution of accidents at work to the workload of the department and to estimate risks of injury in different industrial sectors. Work related injuries accounted for 16.5% of new patients attending the general accident department and 21.7% of those attending eye casualty. Their analysis by industrial sector led to estimates that almost one in 10 workers employed in manufacturing industries and in agriculture, forestry, and fishing attend casualty in the course of a year for a work-related injury. The relatively low risk service sector, because of the large numbers of people employed, contributes the greatest number of individuals with work related injuries. Two industries were identified with very high rates of specific and preventable injuries: food and fish processing, with estimates of 17 knife lacerations per 1000 workers per annum and mechanical engineering with 60 eye injuries per 1000 workers per annum.

Railway accidents receive a great deal of media attention on the few occasions when large numbers of the public are involved. Following the recent series of accidents in the UK there was much discussion as to whether railways were becoming more dangerous. Shepherd and Marshall (1990) studied trends in accidents to railway staff over a 33 year period, 1954–86, which covered the periods pre- and post-modernization of the railways, in conjunction with large reductions in both staffing and traffic volume.

They reported that the Railway Inspectorate, which has the duty of investigating and reporting on accidents occurring on railway premises, defines three kinds of accident: train, movement and non-movement. The number of railway staff killed and injured in each kind of accident was studied in relation to the number of staff employed and train-miles run. Trends in the three accident rates derived thereby showed quite different patterns: for most of the period under study, train accident rates showed a linear increase and movement accident rates a linear decrease, whilst non-movement accidents exhibited no particular trend at all. In the last several years, however, both movement and non-movement accident rates have decreased sharply, whilst train accident rates have increased above the generally rising trend.

CARDIOVASCULAR SYSTEM

The high overall risk of ischaemic heart disease in the United Kingdom has prompted much research in this field to determine if work factors represent additional risks and to determine whether preventive initiatives in the workplace are effective. A study by Deacon (1991) in which workers were offered screening for coronary risk factors (cholesterol, body mass index, blood pressure and smoking habits) had a high uptake, with just over 80% of employees attending voluntarily. Only just over 4% of employees declined to attend, giving the reason that they did not wish to have a health assessment performed; the remaining employees were unable to attend for other reasons, such as work commitments, holidays and sickness absence. The high uptake rate confirms the advantage of workplace based screening. As demonstrated previously, men were shown to have a higher rate of risk factors than women, with high cholesterol, obesity and smoking being the most prevalent risk factors. Cholesterol and blood pressure were demonstrated to increase with increasing body weight. The study concluded that body weight reduction and smoking cessation were the preferred intervention strategies in the occupational health setting. This study did not conclude that serum cholesterol measurements were appropriate in the workplace, although the availability of desk-top analysers now makes this an easy and quick procedure. However, these machines need to be properly operated by well-trained personnel, and the results obtained need careful assessment for their significance. Bhatnagar and Durrington (1993) reported a study in which 94 consecutive patients had serum cholesterol measured by both a desk-top analyser and a hospital laboratory and the results compared. On average, the desk-top analyser reported cholesterol levels 0.6 mmol/l lower than those obtained by the hospital laboratory. The accuracy of the results obtained with the desk-top machine was also influenced by the operator, with accuracy and precision lower when the machine was operated by a nurse than when operated by a laboratory technician. This was despite the fact that the nurse had attended a three-day training course in the use of the machine.

Another study by Majeed et al. (1993) reported a study of 352 measurements by desk-top analyser with simultaneous hospital laboratory analysis. This again reported that the desk-top machine had a negative bias compared with the laboratory one, the mean difference between the two methods of measurement being -0.21 mmol/l, with 95% of the differences lying in the range of 0.95 mmol/l below to 0.52 mmol/l above the laboratory result. This study concluded that while the desktop machine was too imprecise to give accurate measures of serum cholesterol, it was acceptable as a screening device, if a suitable level of result from the desk-top machine was chosen, above which a further sample from the patient would be sent for confirmatory testing at a hospital laboratory.

While these papers addressed the technical aspects of measuring cholesterol, others have expressed concern that reducing serum cholesterol, while reducing the risk of coronary heart disease markedly, has led to an increase in 'non-illness' deaths, resulting in the overall death rate remaining the same, with just the cause of death changing.

Bursey (1992) investigated the correlation between serum cholesterol and the occurrence of occupational accidents at the British Nuclear Fuels operation at Sellafield. Over a three-month period, all men between 40 and 50 years of age presenting for their annual medical were offered a comprehensive medical assessment, which included a measurement of serum cholesterol. A total of 410 men were included in this study and their record of factory accidents over the previous two years was investigated. The severity of accidents was graded into those leading to a loss of time at work and those which did not. Analysis showed no significant difference between the mean cholesterol levels in those reporting accidents and those who did not. Neither was there any significant difference in the cholesterol levels of those men who had sustained an accident severe enough to lose time at work. Thus this study did not demonstrate any correlation between cholesterol levels and accidents in this occupational group.

Although there has been much publicity concerning the correlation between increased cholesterol and increased risk of coronary heart disease, there are other risk factors of equal significance. High blood pressure is one such factor, and it is known that salt intake can influence blood pressure in susceptible people. A study was reported by O'Sullivan and Parker (1992), in which the blood pressures of workers in a salt mine were monitored. This study resulted from the concern expressed by the employees that their work may cause high blood pressure and contribute to their cardiovascular risks. This study found that blood pressure levels in the working group were not raised in comparison with those of a control group of workers not occupationally exposed to salt.

It has been estimated that approximately one-fifth of the workforce in industrial societies is employed in shift work. Bursey (1990) did not demonstrate any correlation between shift work and risk of coronary heart disease when he compared 57 shift workers with day worker controls, matched for age, cigarette smoking habits and work status. The recognized risk factors of coronary heart disease of blood pressure, body mass index and random serum cholesterol were compared between the two groups. None of the investigations showed a statistically significant difference between them, and this report supports previous studies that failed to show conclusive evidence of an adverse effect of shift work on the cardiovascular system.

For those employees suffering from coronary heart disease, there is now the increasing opportunity of treatment by coronary artery bypass grafting. Munro (1990) reported a study of 79 male Post Office employees undergoing coronary artery bypass grafting in a two-year period. Nearly 80% were able to resume work within six months of operation and by the end of the follow-up period 65% of them were still working, the majority in their normal employment. Prior to operation, fewer than 30% had been able to work normally. Return to normal work was found to be more likely in younger employees and in those who had either worked up until surgery or who had only had a short length of time away from work prior to surgery. The type of work was also studied. The differences in return to work could not be related to the physical demands of the job, and it was thought that motivation and socioeconomic factors may have accounted for the differences in return to work.

DERMATOLOGY

The increasing use by high-tech industry of clean rooms leads to a larger number of persons working in such environments, with the potential for the emergence of syndromes associated with those working conditions. It is not uncommon for clean rooms to be maintained at a low humidity. Guest (1991) reported a study of employees working in such an environment compared with those working in a natural factory environment. A greater prevalence of symptoms of itching of the face, redness and urticaria was demonstrated in the low humidity exposed workforce. The previous study demonstrated the hazards of working in a clean environment. A study by Ashworth *et al.* (1993) reported that a problem of chronic irritant contact dermatitis occurring in a group of airline employees working in a warehouse demonstrated the cause of the problem to be over-frequent hand washing, as they had a heightened perception of the risk of skin disease from handling aircraft parts. This research demonstrated that in trying to protect themselves, the employees had caused the problem they were trying to avoid.

DIABETES

People with diabetes may be discriminated against when seeking work as potential employers may feel that they are more likely to lose time from work due to sickness or that their condition will deteriorate and lead to premature retirement on medical grounds. Poole *et al.* (1994) compared the absence rates of a group of diabetic employees in a large engineering factory with a group of non diabetic employees in the same factory, matched for age, sex and occupation. Although the sickness absence was greater in the diabetic group, the mean sickness for diabetics being approximately 50% worse than for non diabetics, the large variability in the sickness absence in both diabetic and non diabetic employees made it impossible to prove this statistically.

The effect of shift work on diabetes was also investigated by Poole *et al.* (1992). Up until 1982 avoidance of shift work was supported by the British Diabetic Association on the grounds that irregular hours made it more difficult to establish good diabetic control. With the development of modern insulin regimes, and better technology for easily measuring blood glucose this view has been revised. A prospective study of diabetics, working either regular days or shifts in a large car assembly plant was undertaken. The results indicated that diabetic control was poor in these workers, whether they were on shifts or regular days. Those subjects who moved to a more rapidly rotating shift pattern demonstrated a significant deterioration in their diabetic control. The conclusion was drawn that there was no difference in the degree of diabetic control achieved between regular day work and slowly rotating shift patterns.

Waclawski (1991a) investigated whether better control of diabetes lead to a decrease in sickness absence in diabetic workers attending a Scottish diabetic clinic. The patients were employed in a number of different industries. The degree of diabetic control was assessed by measuring the level of glycosylated haemaglobin, an objective test which gives an indication of the integrated value of the degree of recent diabetic control. On the basis of this test result the patients were split into two groups, those with good control and those with poor control. The poorly controlled group had statistically significant worse sickness absence records than those with good control, indicating that efforts to increase their level of control could reduce their sickness absence rates.

Waclawski (1991b) further investigated the effects of diabetes on ill health in early retirement by looking at all cases of medical retirement in one year of local government employees in one area. The prevalence of diabetes amongst the retiring group was approximately six times that expected from population studies. Approximately 40% of the diabetics retiring were doing so on the grounds of diabetes or diabetic complications, 30% were retiring for diabetes and other pathology and in only just over 25% was diabetes an incidental factor to other pathology. This indicates that morbidity from diabetes, as assessed by premature medical retirement, is greater than expected.

EAR NOSE AND THROAT

Many workplaces have hearing conservation programmes, often including regular audiometry. McBride (1993) reported a study in the mining industry, which assessed the validity of a self-administered hearing questionnaire in the assessment of risk to hearing. The study concluded that a questionnaire could be used to document hearing loss risk factors, but that it was not a useful tool to detect ear disease.

Whilst noise damage to hearing is well documented, the risk of injury to ears in some industries is not well documented, although recognized by those directly involved. Fisher and Gardiner (1991) reported on the risk of injury to ears in welders, the principal agent of damage being hot metal sparks which can reach temperatures of over 1000°C. They reported on a series of five patients with various severities of injuries and commented on the inadequate ear protection afforded by conventional safety helmets.

INFECTION

Several researchers have investigated hepatitis B infection, particularly in relation to emergency services personnel. This represents the increasing awareness of employers and employees of the potential for infection and the availability of vaccine to protect workers from these risks. Springbett et al. (1994) reported a survey of 472 Gloucestershire firemen who had occupational exposure to blood and body fluids.

Only two people (0.42%) showed evidence of hepatitis B infection. This compares with a 0.49% rate found in a recent study of UK blood donors. Thus an occupational risk of hepatitis B infection was not found in this group, despite considerable occupational exposure to blood and body fluids.

Lancashire ambulance personnel were studied by Morgan-Capner and Wallice (1990), who reported that 1.1% of emergency ambulance personnel showed evidence of past hepatitis B infection, with none showing current infection.

A similar survey of local authority employees working with children or in the community with physically and mentally disabled individuals, reported by Kudesia et al. (1993), showed a prevalence of hepatitis B infection of 1.2%. This was not significantly different from previously reported figures of the prevalence in blood donor groups. Of interest, however, is that 80% of those people identified as having past hepatitis B infection were those who had been in long-term institutional care.

Astbury and Baxter (1990) reported on a study of 1800 clinical health care staff, which showed an overall sharps injury rate of 116 injuries per 100 staff per year. Despite the professional knowledge of this group, only 24% had received a full course of hepatitis B vaccine, although half of the non-vaccinated people reported that they either were planning to have, or were in the process of receiving, a course of vaccinations. Surgical procedures were the commonest cause of accidental injury, accounting for 58% of the total, with the injury rate amongst registrars being 403 injuries per 100 staff per year. Injuries caused by bites and scratches from patients occurred mainly in nurses and auxiliaries in psychiatric geriatric wards, with an injury rate of 115 per 100 staff per year. This demonstrates that despite knowledge about and the availability of vaccination, people at risk do not avail themselves of the service. The most commonly reported reason for not being vaccinated was lack of information about the vaccine.

In a separate study by Gompertz (1990) of medical students, an overall needlestick injury rate of 113 per 100 students per annum was reported, supporting the above mentioned level of injury rate. These studies demonstrated that previously reported needlestick injury rates for hospital personnel of between 6 and 7 injuries per 100 employees (Collins and Kennedy, 1987) underestimate the level of risk. Despite demonstrating the levels of risk for health care employees of injuries which carry the risk of hepatitis B infection, the resource implications for implementing an effective hepatitis B vaccination programme are not always fully realized. Jachuck et al. (1990) demonstrated that to fully implement a vaccination programme for 1000 employees required 4000 additional consultations, necessitating 16 additional hours of occupational health commitment per week. They went on to suggest that Department of Health guidance in implementing vaccination plans should be more specific and should describe the commitment health authorities must make to include appropriate resources to support vaccination programmes.

The problem of educating health care workers about the risk of blood borne infection was investigated by McKinnon et al. (1990), who surveyed hospital workers about their perception of risk and in particular their knowledge and attitudes towards HIV and AIDS problems. As would be expected, clinical workers showed greater knowledge than non-clinical workers. Following the distribution of an information booklet to all the health authority staff, a further survey was undertaken, which demonstrated an improvement in the level of knowledge and a reduction in the level of perceived risk. The greatest improvement was demonstrated in those persons who initially had the least level of knowledge. It is important to consider all health care workers to be potentially at risk from sharps injuries. Williams (1993), in an anonymous survey of hospital hygiene service engineers, reported that over half reported finding sharp objects, including needles, in the washrooms in which they worked, with 23% reporting that this was a frequent occurrence. This survey also demonstrated that a significant number of sharps injury accidents were not being reported.

MUSCULO-SKELETAL

There has been much debate as to whether repetitive strain injury (RSI) exists as a clinical entity or not, with conflicting expert opinions given and inconsistent court judgments. The use of the term has been criticized as being inaccurate, and the use of the term 'upper limb disorder' has been suggested as an alternative. However, Pheasant (1992) was of the opinion that RSI did exist, even if the label was unfortunate, and that it applied to a wide range of clinical states, some of which were more fully understood than others. Patently, more research into this area is required.

Chatterjee (1992) reported an eight-year prospective study into the occurrence of upper limb disorder in an electro-mechanical production plant. During the course of the study remedial action was taken to reduce the risks, when specific causative factors were identified. The condition was shown to occur more frequently in women than in men, with no significant differences between the ages of the affected and non-affected people. Ergonomic study of the jobs indicated three main areas of concern. These were sitting, reach (particularly the interaction between small female operatives and machinery which was too big for them) and posture. Job analysis showed that the repetitive jobs were of the highest risk, with 25 000 hand motions required during each work shift. Prompt reporting of symptoms, with rapid engineering modifications to correct ergonomic and other risk factors, promoted speedy recovery from the condition and immediately reduced the incidence of new cases associated with that task.

Bonsall *et al.* (1991) reported on a study to test the effect of an occupational physiotherapy service on absence attributed to sickness. No effect on total sickness absence rates was demonstrated, although there was possibly an improvement in short-term sickness absence rates. It was noted that a change in management attitude to absence caused a significant reduction in short-term sickness absence rates, confirming the old adage that short-term sickness absence is a management rather than a medical problem.

Back injuries are some of the most frequent occupational injuries, and hospitals have a higher incidence than most other places of work. Turnbull *et al.* (1992) surveyed a 10% sample of the employees of a district health authority and discovered that over half of the respondents had suffered significant spinal pain in the last year. This prompted action to implement a programme to reduce the number and severity of back problems occurring to their employees. However, the real problem is knowing what programmes to implement.

The Manual Handling Regulations, recently introduced to bring the United Kingdom into line with Europe, aim to reduce the most commonly seen adverse effect of manual handling, that is back pain. Smedley and Coggon (1994) reviewed the extensive literature on the subject and concluded that the legislation was based on sound scientific principles. It was recognized that work with a bent or twisted posture, and lifting or carrying heavy loads, carries a high risk of back injury. However, the proposed preventive strategies are largely theoretical and unproven. In particular, the results of training workers in methods of safe manual handling have proved disappointing and more research is required to develop strategies that demonstrably reduce the morbidity from this common problem.

The problem of lack of knowledge about the effects of primary preventive strategies, indicating a need for further research, is not just a European issue. Spitzer (1993) came to a similar conclusion in his review of Canadian practice.

OPHTHALMOLOGY

The recent introduction in the United Kindom of the Display Screen Equipment Regulations has prompted interest in the problems of visual acuity with reference to display screen equipment, in particular visual display units.

Silver and Daniel (1992) reported a study of 103 display screen equipment users, only eight of whom complained of any visual difficulties whilst working with display screen equipment. Interestingly, half of the sample population were using their display screen equipment at, or close to, the normal reading distance, not the intermediate distance often quoted. Only four persons of the total group were found to need visual correction specifically for the display screen distance. They also suggested that even with the advent of lap-top and notebook computers, with the screens both closer and lower than standard personal computers and terminals, the use of normal reading or multifocal prescriptions gives adequate visual acuity.

Occupational eye injury is a constant source of concern especially in the chemical industry. Griffith and Jones (1994) published a study of 62 839 workers in the chemical industry. The observations were taken over one month, approximately 10 million man hours, in which 60 eye injuries (45.1% of all eye injuries) were caused by chemicals (eye injury incidence 11.4 per 1000 employees per year). Six people required hospital attention and no sight threatening injuries occurred. These authors feel that health workers within the industry have recognized that most of these injuries are avoidable. However eye protectors were not a requirement in some situations where injury occurred (one-third of injuries). In some cases eye protection was not used where specified, and in others eye protection failed to prevent injury even when worn. The authors concluded the report by suggesting that this low incidence of injury can be reduced further by appropriate selection and wearing of protectors, by education and by legislation.

Colour perception requirements vary in different jobs and can be critical in certain industries such as aviation and electrical. McElearney, Waddy and Rawll (1992) undertook a study in pre-employment colour vision testing. One thousand and twenty male candidates for employment in occupations that require discrimination of colour were subjected to the Ishihara test and two trade tests of colour perception, the Giles Archer Lantern test and the Electricity Supply Industry (IES) wire test. One hundred candidates failed the Ishihara test, 61 of the 100 passed both trade tests; 16 of the 100 passed the wire test alone and seven of the 100 passed the lantern test alone but only 16 failed all three tests. Seventy-seven of the 84 who passed some part of their colour perception assessment were offered employment appropriate to their colour vision ability. Eleven of the 16 who passed the wire test alone and three of the six who passed the lantern test alone successfully entered employment. Clearly, the Ishihara test, whilst being a useful screening test, is not sufficient on its own as a test of suitability for employment; one or more trade tests should be administered before rejecting candidates who fail it.

PRE-EMPLOYMENT MEDICAL ASSESSMENT

Pre-employment medical assessment is carried out in many different ways, but whether there is any value in this to the employee or prospective employer is sometimes questioned. Some screening procedures are arguably performed for historical rather than good scientific reasons. Chaturvedi and Cockcroft (1992) reviewed the need for pre-employment screening in health service employees to exclude tuberculosis. Retrospective analysis of pre-employment chest X-ray and tuberculin skin test status was undertaken for employees of a health district. It was concluded that X-ray abnormalities were rare and were not predicted by testing tuberculin skin reactivity. Neither procedure was justified as a routine means of screening for tuberculosis in the study population, although the authors conceded that this situation may be different in districts with a high incidence of tuberculosis.

Evans and Aw (1992) reviewed the results of pre-employment haematological screening in almost 1000 employees of a Midlands health authority. Although many abnormalities were found, few were judged to be clinically significant and in only one case did the result affect employment. Again, this method of screening was deemed to be an unnecessary part of pre-employment screening for National Health Service employees.

Braddick, Atwell and Aw (1992) audited the pre-employment health assessment carried out in 17 different occupational health departments within one health authority. They documented a wide variation in practice and commented that a more selective approach to pre-employment procedures could be adopted, with subsequent savings of a significant amount of occupational health staff time.

RESPIRATORY

Meredith, Taylor and McDonald (1991) reported on the work of the SWORD project group, a voluntary scheme for the surveillance of work related and occupational respiratory disease established in January 1989 with help from the British Thoracic Society and the Society of Occupational Medicine and support from the Health and Safety Executive in the UK. Three hundred and fifty-four chest physicians representing 90% of the chest clinics in the UK and 361 occupational physicians regularly submit reports of newly diagnosed cases of work related respiratory illness with information on age, sex, residence, occupation, and suspected causal agent. In 1989, 2101 cases were notified, of which frequent diagnoses were asthma (26%), mesothelioma (16%), pneumoconiosis (15%), benign pleural disease (11%), and allergic alveolitis (6%). Incidence rates calculated against denominators from the Labour Force Survey showed very large differences between occupational groups, especially for asthma and asbestos-related diseases. Substantial regional variation in the incidence of asthma was not explained by the geographical distribution of high risk industries and was probably due to differing levels of ascertainment. The results imply that the true frequency of acute occupational respiratory disease in the UK may have been three times greater than that reported.

The incidence of occupational asthma is apparently rising, due to a combination of increased awareness of the problem and increasing exposure to known sensitizing agents, such as isocyanates. The Midland Thoracic Society's Rare Respiratory Disease Registry Surveillance Scheme of Occupational Asthma (SHIELD) is confined to occupational asthma alone occurring in the West Midlands Region. This scheme collects more detailed information on individual cases than the SWORD scheme. Gannon and Sherwood Burge (1993) reported the results of the scheme and demonstrated an incidence of 43 new cases per million general workers per year. Specific and occupational incidence varied from 1833 per million paint sprayers to 8 per million clerks. They commented that the recognized incidence of occupational asthma is likely to be an underestimate of the true incidence.

Economic factors play their part in this under-reporting, as demonstrated by Gannon et al. (1993), who demonstrated that 32% of patients diagnosed as suffering from occupational asthma remained exposed to the causative agent more than one year after initial diagnosis despite their increasing symptoms and deterioration in lung function. This contrasted with those who had been removed from exposure, in which group there were fewer respiratory symptoms, and whose lung function had improved although they were worse off financially, with a median loss of 54% of annual income. This demonstrates that early diagnosis and removal from exposure is important for improvement in the condition but that inadequate compensation may contribute to the worker deciding to remain exposed, despite its adverse health effect.

The exact cause of occupational asthma is still unknown. Agius et al. (1994) looked at low molecular weight substances causing occupational asthma and concluded that there were significantly more reactive groups in the active chemicals than in a control group of chemicals selected from a list of occupational exposure limits. It is suggested that further study of this area could yield information on the causation of the condition and help in hazard assessment of novel chemical compounds.

Not all exposure to sensitizing agents leads to occupational asthma. Gatley (1991) reported on chiropodists exposed to human nail dust. It was confirmed that sensitization to trichophytons (fungi which infected nails) was common but it did not produce chest symptoms, and no cases of occupational asthma were discovered although allergic upper respiratory tract symptoms were common.

The current methods of detection of occupational asthma amongst workforces are the use of respiratory symptom questionnaires and lung function monitoring, although the sensitivity and specificity of these measures has been questioned. Stenton *et al.* (1993) reported a study of shipyard workers, where the results of questionnaires and lung function were compared against the results of airway responsiveness to inhaled methacholine (a measure of asthmatic potential). The results demonstrated that both questionnaire and lung function measurements had a low sensitivity for detecting possible asthmatic activity and that caution should be exercised when introducing these results to make a diagnosis of occupational asthma amongst the working population.

Chinn *et al.* (1993) looked at the problems of interpreting lung function results from the age of 16 as a guide to lung function in adult life. In assessment of occupational lung effects the results of lung function tests before and after some years of occupational exposure are compared, the difference between the two taken to represent the ages at the times of measurement, the occupational and medical history, the exposure to tobacco smoke and the variability of the measurements. The age of first measurement should preferably be after that at which lung function has attained the adult value; the subsequent decline can then be compared with the longitudinal reference value. Age 25 is usually taken as the average for attaining adult values, but in some industries no measurement is taken at this age, although lung function may have been made at the first pre-employment examination at the age of 16.

To determine whether this result could be used reliably the lung function of shipyard apprentices was assessed from entry in their 17th year to age 25 or 27. The study concluded that the ideal first measurement on which to base estimates of longitudinal decline in lung function was one taken at age 25, but that those taken at 16 could be used instead, and that where such results were available they should not be discounted.

Seaton and Wales (1994) reported on an eight-year follow-up of workers potentially exposed to *Aspergillus niger*, a weak antigen in the manufacture of citrus acid. They demonstrated that reducing exposure with engineering controls was effective in preventing new cases of occupational asthma and that exclusion of potential new workers with positive skin test reactions to *Aspergillus niger* was not necessary.

Various inhalation agents have been responsible for respiratory disease. Schilling and Schilling (1991) reported chest X-ray screening for lung cancer at three UK chromate plants from 1955 to 1989. Chest X-ray screening for lung cancer had been undertaken over a period of 34 years, initially at yearly intervals, then at eight-monthly intervals, on chromate workers at three plants in the UK. A review of the records of 229 employees who were diagnosed as having carcinoma of the lung during the screening programme was conducted. Survival data were available on 124 cases. The cases were analysed by age and regularity of attendance for screening. The numbers detected by works X-ray screening and by other means were determined with five and 10 year survival rates. A modest but predictable improvement in the five year survival of those who attended regularly for radiography was shown. Taking the total population of cases for whom screening was available, no significant improvement in five year survival was found.

Davies, Easton and Bidstrup (1991) also reported on the mortality from respiratory cancer and other causes in UK chromate production workers. Their report updates a 1981 study of mortality at three chromate producing factories and pays special attention to workers engaged after major plant and process changes were completed during 1958–60. The study covered 2298 payroll workers in post on 1st January 1950 or entering employment up to 30th June 1976 and remaining at least one year, with mortality observed up to 31st December 1988. Expected numbers of deaths were calculated from national death rates adjusted for social class and area differences. At the two largest factories 1422 men starting work before the process changes showed a highly significant excess of deaths from lung cancer. They also had a significant excess of deaths from nasal cancer; the four affected men all had over 20 years of employment. Six hundred and seventy-seven men starting work after the completion of process changes showed no excess of lung cancer deaths but the possibility of the risk persisting at a reduced level cannot be excluded. The risk among earlier entrants affected men with two or more years of employment and was highest among those working for 10 years or longer. The relative risk was already raised 4–14 years after first employment; it was highest in the 25–40 year period, but was still raised 50 years after first exposure. The risk showed most clearly at young ages. The excess was greater among men in jobs with high exposure to chromates than among men in less exposed jobs. Less evidence of a lung cancer excess was found among 199 men employed at a third small factory. No risk was apparent in further groups of 214 salaried works staff or 95 workers at an adjacent fertilizer plant. No significant excesses of deaths from cancers of other sites were found.

Gardiner et al. (1993) studied the respiratory health effects of carbon black. A study population of 3086 employees was identified in 18 carbon black production plants in seven European countries. Respiratory health questionnaires, spirometry and chest radiographs were used to estimate effects on health, and personal monitoring procedures were employed to measure current exposure to inspirable and respirable dust along with sulphur and carbon monoxide. The low concentrations of gaseous contaminants made the generation of their current and cumulative exposure indices impossible. Low responses from some plants restricted the final analysis to 1742 employees in 15 plants (81% response rate) for respiratory symptoms and spirometry, and 1096 chest radiographs from 10 plants (74% response rate). In total, 1298 respirable and 1317 inspirable dust samples as well as 1301 sulphur dioxide and 1322 carbon monoxide samples were collected. This study was the first to include a comprehensive and concurrent assessment of occupational exposure to carbon black dust and its associated gaseous contaminants. Cough, sputum and the symptoms of chronic bronchitis were found to be associated with increasing indices of current exposure. Lung function tests also showed small decreases in relation to increasing dust exposure in both smokers and non-smokers. Nearly 25% of the chest radiographs showed small opacities of category 0/1 or greater. These were strongly associated with indices of cumulative dust exposure. The findings are consistent with a non-irritant effect of carbon black dust on the airways combined with dust retention in the lungs.

Sheikh and Guest (1990) reported on respiratory ill health in dental laboratory technicians by a comparative study of doctor consultation rates. They observed that these technicians were nearly three times more likely to consult their doctor with respiratory problems than members of a control group, and 1.7 times more likely to see their doctor with other problems. There was a higher prevalence of continuing bronchospasm in the technician group as evidenced by their increased level of use of bronchodilator therapy.

Thomas et al. (1991) studied factors relating to the development of respiratory symptoms in coffee process workers after several cases of occupational asthma had been reported in a coffee processing factory in England. One hundred and ninety-seven coffee workers, representing 80% of the production workforce, were studied to determine the factors effecting the development of work related respiratory symptoms of wheeze cough and dyspnoea. Respiratory questionnaires and skin prick tests were used. The study concluded that castor bean extract contamination remains a potential problem in the coffee processing industry.

One case of asthma caused by exposure at work to EPO 60, an epoxy resin hardening agent, was reported by Lambourn et al. (1992). Inhalation tests with the hardening agent and resin reproducibly produced an isolated late asthmatic response without change in airway responsiveness to inhaled histamine.

STRESS

Cox (1994) identified factors in the workplace which are now commonly agreed to have the potential to cause stress. These include not only physical factors such as heat and noise, but also pressures caused by the way work is organized and managed. The review argues that a systematic and problem solving approach, based on employees assessing risks and taking sensible practicable steps to remove or minimize them, could usefully be applied to occupational stress as well as other workplace hazards. Although more research is still needed on some aspects of occupational stress, enough is now known to enable practical guidance to be drawn up to help employers identify and tackle the problem in the workplace. This is one of the main conclusions of Cox's work.

Following recent disasters, post-traumatic stress has become accepted as a known effect of the incidents on some individuals. A review by Fraser (1991) of the effects of the Piper Alpha disaster on Grampian police force personnel involved in the incident recorded that potential psychological ill health had been reduced by many factors. These included good management, recognition of the potential problem, liaison with outside agencies, public awareness and support, adequate briefing, time to prepare, visits from senior management and by mental health consultants and occupational health staff, and a follow-up stress questionnaire to identify any ongoing problems. At the time of his report, there was no evidence of ongoing post-traumatic stress disorder in the Grampian police force as a result of involvement in the Piper Alpha disaster.

McCloy (1992) recognized that management of Fire Service personnel should start immediately after traumatic events with debriefing and peer group support of participants in the incidents. For those continuing to experience symptoms after the first week, referral to occupational health advisers or general practitioners was required, and if this did not alleviate the symptoms, referral to specialists was required. She was of the opinion that the most important factor in the treatment of the condition was to acknowledge its existence in the first place.

Other stressful incidents occurring at work can have an effect on the individual's psychological health. Jenkinson (1993) reported on a study of over 200 postmen attacked whilst on duty in Northern Ireland over a four-year period, in which the pattern of absences due to psychological causes for the six months after the attack was analysed. Armed attacks produced significantly more frequent and longer episodes of absence, whereas the incidence of absence after only violent attacks was not significantly greater, although when absence occurred it was for a longer period. Approximately 10% of the group were unfortunate enough to sustain a second attack during the study period, and in these there was a fivefold increase in the length of sickness absence taken after the second attack.

Research has demonstrated that some potentially stressful work situations do not produce any demonstrable effect. Gann, Corpe and Wilson (1990) reported on a study of offshore oil workers in the North Sea. Despite the hazardous environment, no difference was demonstrated in anxiety and depression scores using a Goldberg questionnaire (Goldberg *et al.*, 1988), compared with a control group of onshore workers.

SUMMARY

Research in occupational health is abundant and clearly not all the issues are addressed here. However, it appears that research in occupational health, despite the organizational problems, is currently addressing some of the issues highlighted by the Labour Force Survey.

Harrington (1994), using a survey questioning 53 senior practitioners of occupational medicine, canvassed views on resources for research priorities in occupational medicine in the United Kindom. There was a high response rate of 86%. The first priority was for more research on the natural history of work related ill health, specifically identifying musculo-skeletal disorders of the back and upper limbs, followed by asthma, accidents, skin disorders, vibration induced disease, suicide and depression, and finally hearing loss. The second priority area was audit, particularly for its use in occupational health screening procedures. The environmental impact of industrial activity was the third priority, with stress-related disease, with particular emphasis on risk factors, being the fourth priority. The fifth priority was neuropsychological effects of work exposure, and in particular the need for more research on diagnostic tests. Other areas of concern identified were the cost effectiveness of occupational health, risk assessment, reproductive hazards, the effects of pharmacological agents and the development of biomarkers as early evidence of an exposure effect.

As long as people are employed, interest in research into occupational health will continue.

REFERENCES

Agius, R.M., Elton, R.A., Sawyer, L. and Taylor, P. (1994) Occupational asthma and the chemical properties of low molecular weight organic substances. *Occupational Medicine*, **44**, 34–6.

Ashworth, J., Rycroft, R.J.G., Waddy, R.S. and Irvine, D. (1993) Irritant contact dermatitis in warehouse employees. *Occupational Medicine*, **43**, 32–4.

Astbury, C. and Baxter, P.J. (1990) Infection risks in hospital staff from blood: hazardous injury rates and acceptance of hepatitis B immunization. *Journal of the Society of Occupational Medicine*, **40**, 92–3.

Baxter, P.J. (1991) Research in occupational health: the U.K. National Health Service. *Journal of the Society of Occupational Medicine*, **41**, 7–9.

Bhatnagar, D. and Durrington, P.N. (1993) An evaluation of the Reflotron for the determination of plasma cholesterol in capillary blood. Effect of operator variability. *Occupational Medicine*, **43**, 69–72.

Bonsall, J.J., Squier, J.E.O., Baron, C.A. and Parker, G. (1991) Effect of physiotherapy on sickness absence in industry: a comparative study. *Journal of the Society of Occupational Medicine*, **41**, 176–80.

Braddick, M.R., Atwell, C.P. and Aw, T.C. (1992) Audit of pre-employment health assessment in the National Health Service. *Occupational Medicine*, **42**, 36–8.

Bursey, R.G. (1990) A cardiovascular study of shift workers with respect to coronary artery disease risk factor prevalence. *Journal of the Society of Occupational Medicine*, **40**, 65–7.

Bursey, R.G. (1992) Non-significance of plasma total cholesterol in the occurrence of occupational accidents. *Occupational Medicine*, **42**, 33–5.

Chatterjee, D.S. (1992) Workplace upper limb disorders: A prospective study with intervention. *Occupational Medicine*, **42**, 129–36.

Chaturvedi, N. and Cockcroft, A. (1992) Tuberculosis screening in health service employees: who needs chest X-rays? *Occupational Medicine*, **42**, 179–82.

Chinn, D.J., Cotes, J.E., Fechner, M. and Elliott, C. (1993) Pre-employment lung function at age 16 years as a guide to lung function in adult life. *British Journal of Industrial Medicine*, **50**, 422–7.

Coggon, D. (1990) Occupational health research – Looking to the next decade. *Journal of the Society of Occupational Medicine*, **40**, 38–9.

Collins, C.H. and Kennedy, D.A. (1987) Microbiological hazards of needlestick. *Journal of Applied Bacteriology*, **62**, 385–402.

Cox, T. (1994) Stress research and stress management: putting theory to work. HSE Contract Research Report No. 61/1993, HSE Books, Sudbury, UK.

Davies, J.M., Easton, D.F. and Bidstrup, P.L. (1991) Mortality from respiratory cancer and other causes in United Kingdom chromate production workers. *British Journal of Industrial Medicine*, **48**, 299–313.

Deacon, S.P. (1991) Screening for coronary risk factors in occupational health practice. *Journal of the Society of Occupational Medicine*, **41**, 126–8.

Diamond, P.A.M. (1990) Needs of occupational health practitioners: industrial priorities in next 10 years in transport. *Journal of the Society of Occupational Medicine*, **40**, 129.

Evans, G. and Aw, T.C. (1992) Should prospective NHS employees have routine blood counts? *Occupational Medicine*, **41**, 79–82.

Fisher, E.W. and Gardiner, Q. (1991) Tympanic membrane injury in welders: Is prevention neglected? *Journal of the Society of Occupational Medicine*, **41**, 86–8.

Fraser, D.E. (1991) Occupational health management of police officers involved in the Piper Alpha disaster. *Journal of the Society of Occupational Medicine*, **41**, 174–5.

Gann, M. Corpe, U. and Wilson, I. (1990) The application of a short anxiety and depression questionnaire to oil industry staff. *Journal of the Society of Occupational Medicine*, **40**, 138–42.

Gannon, P.F.G. and Sherwood Burge, P. (1993) The SHIELD scheme in the West Midlands Region, United Kindom. *British Journal of Industrial Medicine*, **50**, 791–6.

Gannon, P.F.G., Weir, D.C., Robertson, A.S. and Sherwood Burge, P. (1993)

Health, employment and financial outcomes in workers with occupational asthma. *British Journal of Industrial Medicine*, **50**, 491–6.

Gardiner, K., Trethowan, N.W., Harrington, J.M. *et al.* (1993) Respiratory health effects of carbon black: a survey of European carbon black workers. *British Journal of Industrial Medicine*, **50**, 1082–96.

Gatley, M. (1991) Human nail dust: hazard to chiropodists or merely nuisance? *Journal of the Society of Occupational Medicine*, **41**, 121–5.

Goldberg, D., Bridges, K., Duncan-Jones, P. and Grayson, D. (1988) Detecting anxiety and depression in general medical settings. *British Medical Journal*, **297**, 897–9.

Gompertz, S. (1990) Needlestick injuries in medical students. *Journal of the Society of Occupational Medicine*, **40**, 19–20.

Griffith, G.A.P. and Jones, N.P. (1994) Eye injury and eye protection: a survey of the chemical industry. *Occupational Medicine*, **44**, 37–40.

Guest, R. (1991) Clean rooms and itchy faces. *Journal of the Society of Occupational Medicine*, **41**, 37–40.

Harker, C., Matheson, A.B., Ross, J.A.S. and Seaton, A. (1991) Accidents in the workplace. *Journal of the Society of Occupational Medicine*, **41**, 73–6.

Harrington, J.M. (1990) Research in occupational medicine – thriving or dying? *Journal of the Society of Occupational Medicine*, **40**, 29–33.

Harrington, J.M. (1994) Research priorities in occupational medicine: a survey of United Kingdom medical opinion by the Delphi technique. *Occupational and Environmental Medicine*, **51**, 289–94.

Heap, D. (1993) The health care industry. *Occupational Medicine*, **43**, 47–50.

Hodgson, J.T., Jones, J.R., Elliott, R.C. and Osman, J. (1993) Self-reported work related illness: results from a trailer questionnaire on the 1990 Labour Force Survey in England and Wales. HSE Research Paper 33, HSE Books, Sudbury, UK.

Jachuck, S.J., Jones, C., Nicholls, A. and Bartlett, M. (1990) Resource needs of an occupational health service to accommodate a hepatitis B vaccination programme. *Journal of the Society of Occupational Medicine*, **40**, 89–91.

Jenkinson, W.R. (1993) Attacks on postmen in Northern Ireland. What features of the attacks are associated with prolonged absence from work? *Occupational Medicine*, **43**, 39–42.

Kudesia, G., Briggs, D., Donaldson M. *et al.* (1993) Hepatitis B prevalence in local authority employees. *Occupational Medicine*, **43**, 129–31.

Lambourn, E.M., Hayes, J.P., McAllister, W.A.C. and Newman Taylor, A.J. (1992) Occupational asthma due to EPO 60. *British Journal of Industrial Medicine*, **49**, 294–5.

McBride, D. (1993) Hearing conservation in the mining industry. Evaluation of a risk factor questionnaire. *Occupational Medicine*, **43**, 185–92.

McCloy, E. (1992) Management of post-incident trauma: a fire service perspective. *Occupational Medicine*, **42**, 163–6.

McElearney, N.L.G., Waddy, R.S. and Rawll, C.C.G. (1992) Pre-employment colour vision testing. *Occupational Medicine*, **42**, 19–22.

McKiernan, M.J. (1990) Research in occupational health: engineering industry perspective. *Journal of the Society of Occupational Medicine*, **40**, 127–8.

McKinnon, M.D., Insall, C., Gooch, C.D. and Cockcroft, A. (1990) Knowledge and attitudes of health care workers about AIDS and HIV infection before and after distribution of an educational booklet. *Journal of the Society of*

Occupational Medicine, **40**, 15–18.

Majeed, F.A., Turner, H.J., Stuart, J.M. *et al.* (1993) Audit of near patient cholesterol testing in occupational health clinics. *Occupational Medicine*, **43**, 23–6.

Meredith, S.K., Taylor, V.M. and McDonald, J.C. (1991) Occupational respiratory disease in the United Kingdom 1989: a report to the British Thoracic Society and the Society of Occupational Medicine by the SWORD project group. *British Journal of Industrial Medicine*, **48**, 292–8.

Morgan-Capner, P. and Wallice, P.D.B. (1990) Hepatitis B markers in ambulance personnel in Lancashire. *Journal of the Society of Occupational Medicine*, **40**, 21–2.

Munro, W.S. (1990) Work before and after coronary artery bypass grafting. *Journal of the Society of Occupational Medicine*, **40**, 59–64.

O'Sullivan, J.J. and Parker, G.D.J. (1992) Investigation of the blood pressure levels of workers occupationally exposed to salt. *Occupational Medicine*, **42**, 15–18.

Pheasant, S.T. (1992) Does RSI exist? *Occupational Medicine*, **42**, 164–8.

Poole, C.J.M., Gibbons, D. and Calvert, I.A. (1994) Sickness absence in diabetic employees at a large engineering factory. *Occupational and Environmental Medicine*, **51**, 299–301.

Poole, C.J.M., Wright, A.D. and Nattrass, M. (1992) Control of diabetes mellitus in shift workers. *British Journal of Industrial Medicine*, **49**, 513–15.

Reporting of Injuries, Diseases and Dangerous Occurrences Regulations 1985 (Statutory Instrument 1985 No. 2023), HMSO, UK.

Schilling, C.J. and Schilling, J.M. (1991) Chest X-ray screening for lung cancer at three British chromates plants from 1955 to 1989. *British Journal of Industrial Medicine*, **48**, 476–9.

Schilling, R.S.F. (1993) A university's contribution to occupational health. *British Journal of Industrial Medicine*, **50**, 418–21.

Seaton, A. and Wales, D. (1994) Clinical reactions to *Aspergillus niger* in a biotechnology plant: an eight year follow up. *Occupational and Environmental Medicine*, **51**, 54–6.

Sheikh, M.E. and Guest, R. (1990) Respiratory ill-health in dental laboratory technicians: a comparative study of GP consultation rates. *Journal of the Society of Occupational Medicine*, **40**, 68–70.

Shepherd, S.J. and Marshall, T. (1990) Safety at work for railway staff in Britain. *Journal of the Society of Occupational Medicine*, **40**, 130–4.

Silver, J.H. and Daniel, R.D. (1992) Assessment for display screen users: a hospital based study. *Occupational Medicine*, **42**, 159–162.

Slovak, A.J.M. (1993) Should atopic employees be excluded from specific occupations? *Occupational Medicine*, **43**, 51–2.

Smedley, J. and Coggon, D. (1994) Will the manual handling regulations reduce the incidence of back disorders? *Occupational Medicine*, **44**, 63–5.

Spitzer, W.O. (1993) Low back pain in the workplace: attainable benefits not attained. *British Journal of Industrial Medicine*, **50**, 385–8.

Springbett, R.J., Cartwright, K.A.V., Watson, B.E. *et al.* (1994) Hepatitis B markers in Gloucestershire firemen. *Occupational Medicine*, **44**, 9–11.

Stenton, S.C., Beach, J.R., Avery, A.J. and Hendrick, D.J. (1993) The value of questionnaires and spirometry in asthma surveillance programmes in the workplace. *Occupational Medicine* **43**, 203–6.

Thomas, K.E., Trigg, C.J., Baxter, P.J. *et al.* (1991) Factors relating to the development of respiratory symptoms in coffee process workers. *British Journal of Industrial Medicine,* **48**, 314–22.

Turnbull, N., Dornan, J., Fletcher, B. and Wilson, S. (1992) Prevalence of spinal pain among the staff of a district health authority. *Occupational Medicine,* **42**, 143–8.

Waclawski, E.R. (1991) Ill-health retirement and diabetes mellitus. *Journal of the Society of Occupational Medicine,* **41**, 80–2.

Waclawski, E.R. (1991) Sickness absence and control of insulin-treated diabetes as assessed by glycosylated haemoglobin. *Journal of the Society of Occupational Medicine,* **41**, 119–20.

Williams, N.R. (1993) Needlestick and sharps injuries in hygiene service engineers. *Occupational Medicine,* **43**, 132–4.

Delivering training and education in occupational health for nurses

11

James Garvey

INTRODUCTION

In a few years time the occupational health nurse (OHN) enters the third millennium, and will continue to face a barrage of stimuli from many quarters that will require him or her to be both professional and competent in the delivery of skills. The educationalists within occupational health (OH) have an important duty to make sure that as educators we meet the needs of industry not just for today but for the many tomorrows that may follow. Will then the OHN be prepared for the future and the demands that will be made on the specialism as we enter an era that promises to be unique in its development?

Perhaps from an educational perspective the beauty of OH is that as a taught discipline its boundaries and content are constantly changing. There is little opportunity to stagnate in the time continuum of OH. On the one hand are such things as EU legislation and its practical implications in the workplace and on the other are the diverse effects of technology and its impact on the practitioner.

With this fluctuating framework abounding, how as educationalists do we ensure that the students of today become the professional occupational health practitioners of tomorrow? The following pages will look at the way in which OH is delivered and review the way in which such courses should aim to meet the training needs of their students. How they are assessed on courses, what the courses deliver and finally a look at what is meant by competency and the need for continuing updating mean that OH courses cannot afford to be static or rigid. In today's ever changing climate there is a need for courses to be both flexible and capable of change. One way of achieving this flexibility is to try to aim for a modularized version of the course syllabus. Modular courses are now fairly commonplace in educational establishments. They enable large sections of course material to be broken down into specific parts which once validated can be credited through the credit and accumulation transfer scheme (CATS) with specific points. This enables students to learn at a pace that is appropriate to their own particular situation at a given time. Students may not always be able to undertake a course of full-time education; financial reasons, family commitments, the advantage of part-time work may be just a few of the many reasons that prevent a long-term commitment to full-time education.

Modularization of courses can help students to feel that they have an element of control over their educational process. They can select specific courses or parts of courses and build up their own personal portfolio working perhaps towards a diploma or degree qualification.

DETERMINING TRAINING NEEDS

The Occupational Health Course at Manchester Metropolitan University (MMU) is divided into three distinct modules.

PRINCIPLES AND PRACTICE OF OCCUPATIONAL HEALTH

Here the student focuses on occupational health nursing and tries to see its relevancy within an overall framework of common core subjects. This module covers the history and development of OH and looks at OH within the nursing profession. Students can critically examine the role and function of the OHN and compare this role with that of others working within the nursing profession and specifically within the multiplicity of roles generated by primary health care teams and the ever growing importance of community care. More widely it considers how industry and commerce in the UK affect occupational health services and students will be shown how to identify the nature of workplace hazards and apply standards for their control. Management skills are an essential part of the OHN's role and therefore relevant topics are based on: managing resources, managing people, team-building skills, management of change, personal development, inter-personal skills, communication and data management.

HEALTH WORK AND MAN

This module covers a well-understood concept of OH in so far as its interrelationship is concerned. Organizational cultures and strategies may exert a direct influence on such interaction and these issues are explored. Additionally the management of the individual or group response to hazards in the working environment is considered in relation to occupational and non-occupational ill health. The content of this module aims to promote a critical awareness of issues which affect the health of people at work. In particular an understanding is required of the physiological and psychological aspects of ill health in order to determine their occupational significance. Many of the practical skills often affiliated to the role of the OHN are taught during this module which help to prepare students for their future role within a clinical setting.

ECOLOGY AND THE GLOBAL ENVIRONMENT

This module is designed to explore the much wider issues contained within the 1978 Declaration of Alma Ata issued by the World Health Organization within 'Health for All by the Year 2000'. Consideration is given to ecological and environmental issues where these impinge on OH. The aim here is to develop in the student a lively sense of awareness and sensitivity to global issues which affect health. Furthermore the module tries to encourage OHNs to realize that they are a force for change and as such should be ready to face up to change within their own environments in order that they might contribute to wider change on a global level. As Brown *et al.* (1993) emphasize '. . . a casual survey of the planet's physical condition shows the costs of burning fossil fuels are rising on many fronts. At some point, the economic costs of deteriorating forests, dying lakes, damaged crops, respiratory illnesses, increasing temperatures, rising sea level and other destructive effects become unacceptably high'. The OHN then cannot afford to be isolated from the global issues that affect our environment, but has much to contribute towards creating a safer and cleaner planet, and must be instrumental in helping to formulate policies that will benefit people today and in the future. Brown *et al.* (1993) try to encourage their readers, and their words are equally applicable to OHNs when they say, 'If we fail to convert our self-destructing economy into one that is environmentally sustainable, future generations will be overwhelmed by environmental degrdation and social disintegration. Simply stated, if our generation does not turn things around, our children may not have the option of doing so.'

Given the above package as just one example of how OH might be presented, does it meet the needs of both the student and more specifically does it meet the needs of industry today? One way of finding this out is to undertake a self-audit and evaluation of course content. The author of this chapter recently undertook research into this specific field of enquiry (Garvey, 1993a). In an attempt to determine training needs the author looked at a total of 72 job descriptions and job advertisements. The aim here was to highlight through a content analysis approach the main elements that were considered indicative and indeed necessary for the post of OHN. From the data analysed the author found a total of 39 main elements that were regularly requested by potential employers. The elements were ranked into groups related to their frequency. Of these 39 elements, two predominated specifically throughout the sample. These were:

- Candidates should possess an RGN background and have completed an OHNC qualification.
- Candidates should be good communicators.

That the candidate should hold the RGN or OHNC qualification was clearly seen in the study. It seemed therefore that based on the sample, industry required qualified nurses, rather than non-nursing personnel, to undertake the duties concerned. It is perhaps worth mentioning at this stage that the study had also introduced the concept of non-nursing personnel undertaking OHN activities. Communication skills were equally prevalent as an employer's requirement and indeed these two areas formulate the very core of the conceptual models used to good effect to explain the role of the OHN, i.e. Hanasaari (Alsten *et al.*, 1988) and the Wilkinson Windmill Models (Wilkinson, 1990). Other elements that ranked highly in the study were as follows:

- a need for knowledge of legislation
- screening skills
- first aid skills
- interpersonal skills
- counselling
- workplace visits
- knowledge of hazards.

In so far as the above elements were concerned, screening and health surveillance are still considered to be important areas requiring the attention of the OHN. It was expected that most job descriptions would carry these features. New ERC guidelines were issued in 1993 and companies are looking for ways to save costs and teach their own first aiders. Usually this function falls to the OHN.

In keeping with teaching and with communication in general, the OHN needs a wide variety of interpersonal skills. The OHN encounters many different people during a working day and the only way in which the service will be promoted will be through sound use of such skills in all quarters. Good counselling techniques and interpersonal skills go hand in hand. Also, by undertaking workplace visits a greater appreciation of hazard and risk in this environment will be acquired. It was encouraging to note from the study that some employers understand the need for such visits – the lifeline of OH.

There were many other elements considered within the study: from rehabilitation to research, confidentiality to promoter of the Occupational Health service. All of the elements enabled the author to compare the elements in the research study with the content of the Occupational Health Nursing course at MMU (Diploma of Higher Education in Community Health (Occupational Health)) – otherwise known as the DipHE – and see which were evident within the syllabus and give additional concentration to areas that might need further input. Not content with knowing what industry expected from the product of the educationalist, i.e. the OHN, the author developed a further research tool (Garvey, 1994) in the format of a questionnaire and asked OHNs, occupational physicians and managers what they thought were the main elements of importance in the DipHE programme. This was an opportunity to ask just how effective the course was for them in their chosen specialism. As Figure 11.1 shows, this study concentrated in the main on sampling from the area of occupational health nursing with only 10.8% of the total cohort, i.e. four respondents, being from a medical/managerial background.

The remaining 33 respondents (89.2%) were all from OHN backgrounds. Any further study would have to encapsulate a more rigorous exploitation of data from all three areas in order that a more balanced perspective could be obtained in relation to the issues being explored. However, for the purpose of determining training needs the ques-

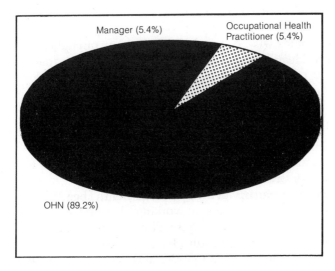

Figure 11.1   Occupation of respondents

tionnaire distribution and analysis was a useful indicator of whether as educationalists we were meeting the needs of our own customers.

In the main the respondents to the questionnaire felt that the course had met their needs and expectations. Respondents, when asked if they thought there were areas of the course content that they would like to see more emphasis on, tended to lean towards the areas of application of practical skills. Many OHNs were concerned that they might be asked to undertake procedures within their specialism that they were not fully trained or competent in; a legitimate concern and one which the course today addresses. So by questioning the students, the recipients of the course, and analysing the needs of industry and equating the two the educationalist is likely to have a better idea of what exactly the needs of his or her specific specialism will require.

Educationalists today cannot afford to be locked away in ivory towers pondering issues which have no meaning or only bare significance in the real world of occupational health. Instead they must be part of the multidisciplinary team constantly working, listening and communicating with those active in the field and capable of producing courses that are relevant to the needs of the specialist.

DELIVERING TRAINING

Applicants for the DipHE in Occupational Health must hold the RGN qualification and have had two years post-registration experience before applying to undertake the course in accordance with English National Board (ENB) directives. After deciding whether to undertake the course on a full-time basis (51 weeks) or on a part-time basis (one day per week for two years), upon successful completion of their chosen course candidates will be awarded the Diploma of Higher Education in Community Health (Occupational Health). The principal aim of the course is to produce a critical practitioner who will develop a person centred approach within a community setting and enhance the current professional role in both a generic and specialist sense.

With this underpinning aim five further general objectives are woven into the course:

(a) To generate critical thought that will enable students to be reflective of their own community practice.
(b) To develop a person centred approach with regard to community health.
(c) To broaden the knowledge base by the understanding and application of explanations of health from various disciplines.
(d) To generate the capacity to offer and receive mentorship, supervision and critical friendship.

(e) To develop skills necessary to enable students to engage in research programmes in health related fields.

The whole emphasis surrounding and underpinning the course is one of flexibility, reflexivity and application.

The DipHE course of study is based on the Health Career Model (HCM) and this has been used for the curricular model. The common core aspect of the DipHE, which includes the subjects of sociology, psychology, social psychology, sociology, sociology of health and illness, social policy, and health promotion, provides the foundation material for the course in a broad sense. The methods of enquiry and evaluation (MEE) facilitate a more focused explanation of these themes and develop a holistic view of health. The HCM has proved to be a useful framework from which to examine other models of care – from the more general biomedical and social models, to the more specific models such as Orem's, Henderson's, Egan's and Hanasaari's. Figure 11.2 illustrates the now familiar Hanasaari model.

HCM does not exclude the student from exploring other models of care, but rather encourages it. Enquiring minds and their development is at the crux of the course. It is interesting to see that two OHNs have already started this process by writing a series of articles on the very

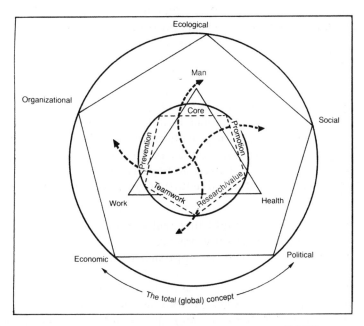

Figure 11.2   The Hanasaari model. Redrawn from Alston (1988).

subject of nursing models. Fairburn and McGettigan (1994) argue that existing occupational health nursing models do not allow for a problem solving approach or challenge established concepts by producing their own model. Whether they would be deemed to be correct or not in assuming that problem solving is not inherent in the models they have looked at is not the issue. What is exciting about the issue is that at last OHNs are taking stock of their professional development and are prepared to challenge and question the major issues that affect their specialism. They state, 'We hope that the model will assist in explaining the unique contribution of the occupational health nurse by outlining the entities and attributes which must be addressed in practice. We consider the way forward to be to work on the development of a model bespoke to the needs of occupational health nursing' (Fairburn and McGettigan, 1994). Here we have a great example of two OHNs prepared to put their skills to good effect.

The OHN at MMU is no longer taught in isolation from other specialisms. The philosophy of greater communication and team work is exemplified though the merging of nine professional branches studying together so that in the future they may work together with a greater knowledge and awareness of each other's skills. The branches are:

- Occupational health nursing
- Learning disabilities
- Community psychiatric nursing
- District nursing
- Health promotion
- Health visiting
- Drugs and alcohol
- School nursing
- Practice nursing

In this way the client groups can benefit from the knowledge that the practitioners working in the community can call upon and utilize relevant expertise as required and that in the end the client will benefit from having a considerable amount of greater choice in the way in which he/she wishes to be cared for. Against this backdrop, and once the needs of training have been ascertained, the educationalist must determine how those needs can be met through the ways in which training can be delivered within and without the educational institution. Above all training or learning needs to be meaningful and relevant. Entering a course of study can be an almost Herculean challenge to the student especially when the student may have responsibilities to his/her employer (if undertaking part-time studies), has to administer to his/her own social and domestic responsibilities and, at the same time, undertake an intensive course of study in OH.

For mature students, facing life as a student again after a long lay off can be a discouraging task in itself. Memories of studying may still be related to 'the school room atmosphere with rows of chairs and teachers at the front of the class imparting wonderful pearls of wisdom which pupils slavishly wrote down and pondered over in so many homework sessions' (Garvey, 1993b).

It can be a strange new scenario for students to cope with when they suddenly realize that learning for them will take on a whole new independent format; that they themselves will be the negotiators through the labyrinth of learning and understanding and that the quality of that experience will fundamentally be of their own making. That isn't to say that the tutor in higher education simply lets the student get on with the task. On the contrary the tutor has a very important role to make sure that this learning curve is traversed effectively and he or she must facilitate the unfolding of these events in order for them to occur. Figure 11.3 illustrates the 'wedge' theory often used to depict the changing roles of tutor/student in academic activity.

As a course commences, as one might expect the role of the tutor is quite dominant. However, as the course continues the role of the tutor starts to decrease and the role of the student continues to increase and he or she develops the skill of being an independent scholar who no longer requires 'spoon-feeding'.

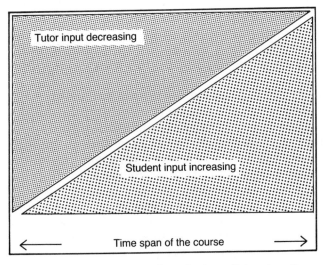

Figure 11.3   The simultaneous changing of roles within education.

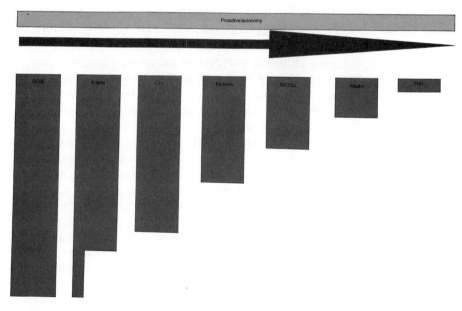

Figure 11.4   The student's route to proactive autonomy.

Figure 11.4 illustrates the development of the student along the proactive autonomous route through education (Garvey, 1994). Here the idea is graphically displayed along the continuum of educational challenges in the format of higher qualifications. The closer we come to the PhD level of education the more we realize our independence, autonomy and level of expertise in the educational setting. Indeed many would agree that this self-awareness and realization is already reached at Diploma level but greater demands are placed on the student to follow this independence and autonomy as higher levels are aspired to.

It is likely that in the not too distant future the specialism of OH will become an all graduate profession.

Many qualified OHNs have already taken steps to upgrade and convert their certificate qualifications to diplomas. The diploma itself will not have a infinite length of time to continue. It is already being overshadowed by degree level courses and soon the basic standard for entry into occupational health nursing will no longer be at diploma level but at degree level and perhaps beyond.

So while students are eagerly trying to obtain their respective qualifications how do the educationalists deliver the quality of material to make the effort worth their while?

In his book on improving student learning, Gibbs (1992) talks about surface and deep approaches to learning. Basically the surface approach would equate with certificate level work that has to be memorized and is assessed by examination. A deep approach takes the information, understands it, focuses a different perspective on it and then tries to apply it and relate it to practice. A student who simply reiterates in an essay what has been given in a lecture or copies word for word information given in a handout is adopting a stringent surface approach that does little to improve the quality of the learner's own scholastic development. The student that can look at, say, an OH issue, e.g. health screening, and relate the concepts and influences of the Hanasaari model to it and develop new perspectives for dealing with the issues and problems is adopting a deeper approach.

Furthermore the quality of learning is improved and there is a sense of achievement in producing a unique and worthwhile piece of work. Gibbs recommends nine strategies for improving the quality of student learning and for fostering a deep approach. These are:

- independent learning
- personal development
- problem-based learning
- reflection
- independent group work
- learning by doing
- developing learning skills
- project work
- fine tuning.

We have already seen the importance of developing independent learning within our students. The independent student today becomes an independent free thinking employee tomorrow capable of making decisions and acting appropriately in the decision-making processes that affect his/her specialism. 'Independent learning involves giving students greater autonomy and control over choice of subject matter, learning methods, pace of study and assessment of learning outcomes' (Gibbs, 1992).

The DipHE programme at MMU tries to foster this independent approach within its curriculum framework which remains flexible to accomodate all individuals.

It is important also to encourage personal development within the timescale of the course. The student who completes a course of study must have changed and developed during the time it has taken to complete and achieve the qualification. If personal development has not taken place one must really question the educational process that students are undertaking. The possibility for students to 'experiment' with the quest for knowledge, its implications, its analysis, synthesis and formulations, and above all the space to be able to reflect on what has been achieved must be to the forefront of the learning domain.

It is only through reflection that advances can be made and that experiences shared and reflected on can actually turn into learning. Gibbs emphasizes that 'methods which encourage reflection include the use of learning diaries, reflective journals and portfolios of work, discussion of learning strategies, specially designed reflective exercises run by lecturers and the use of video, audio and observers in the context of learning which involves performance or behavioural skills' (*op. cit.* p. 14). Reflection is a useful tool in the armoury of decision making. OHNs while students need to use it to its fullest degree so that learning to reflect wisely on their experiences as students enables them to take the same reflective skills with them into their working environments and utilize them with effect in relation to their daily activities, interactions and communications.

Reflection can be utilized when dealing with problem-based learning as a means of acquiring a solution where one is possible. It should be realized that problem-based learning does not by definition imply solutions to problems.

As Gibbs reiterates 'In problem-based learning the problem may not be solvable, but nevertheless provides a rich environment for learning. The aim is to learn rather than solve the problem' (Gibbs, 1992). Activities on the DipHE programme look at real issues from the world of OH and students work together focusing on specific areas, sharing their learning and working in a cooperative team-like manner. Research is one area within the DipHE programme that actively encourages reflection. There are many stages in the research process where the researcher needs to reflect and reflect again on what is being undertaken, e.g. piloting research methodologies is but a way of reflecting if the research process is appropriate to the line of study being undertaken.

Figure 11.5 shows the author's own flow chart strategy and the process involved in action research, from identifying a problem to trying to solve the problem, finding areas of further improvement, and producing suitable findings worthy of publication and sharing with a larger audience; none of these would be possible without the ability to be able to reflect. Indeed reflection time is built into the model strategy. Donald Schon has written two books on the subject (1983, 1987).

Such is the importance of drawing together the idea that, as practitioners in whatever field of employment, we need to reflect in order to grow. Besides encouraging reflection, independent group work, learning by action and developing learning skills are also considered to be fundamental to the delivery of the training package for OHNs.

Students work together on project work, take over the lecturer/tutor

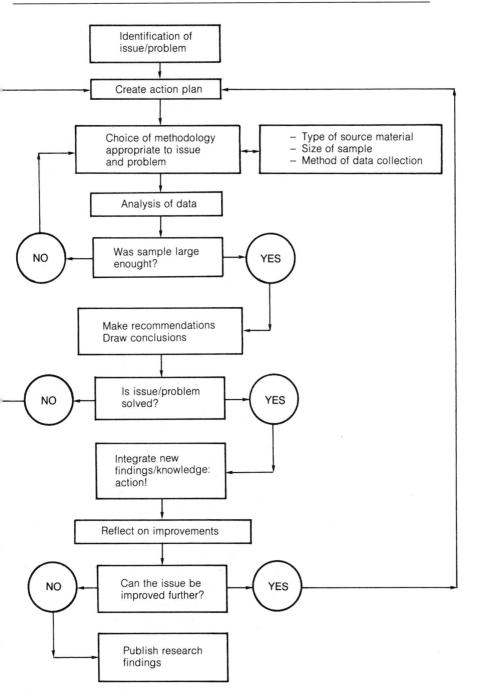

Figure 11.5   Garvey's action research model.

role in student led sessions, and do not just develop intellectual skills but learn practical skills in areas such as audiometry and spirometry. Visits to a wide variety of industrial and commercial enterprises coupled with periods of work experience placements all endeavour to help create additional learning encounters. For the OHNs the culminating piece of evidence that they produce on the course is their project work where the application of knowledge takes on a very practical and tangible format. Most OH projects take the form of environmental surveys. The project allows the OHN student to apply in practice all the theoretical aspects of the course that have been realized and helps to bridge the theory–practice gap with a realistic piece of work that is both beneficial to the student and to the institution that allowed the project to be undertaken. Gibbs (1992) states: 'Project work can be highly motivating for students, capturing a significantly greater proportion of student's time and energy than parallel taught courses of equivalent assessment value. The level of motivation seems to depend on the extent of student's responsibility for choosing and managing the project, and on the extent to which students are involved in negotiating the project's assessment.'

With the advent of trans-cultural nurse education within the field of OH it is now possible, through the network of institutions of higher education (ERASMUS and TEMPUS European funded programmes), to enable student OHNs to travel abroad and undertake project work in cultures and societies other than their own. The challenge that this brings to the students appears to motivate them highly and the work produced is of a very high calibre. As Hodgkinson (1992) states, 'The prime motive is to give UK students educational and cultural opportunities beyond those that exist in the home institution. They are thereby fitted to operate in the wider European employment market. Also, there is little doubt that the presence within the home institution of guest students from a variety of other countries creates opportunities for cultural interaction, which are a benefit to all students and staff.'

Trans-cultural nurse education helps to bring an even greater global dimension to nurse education. The fact that institutions are interested in sharing with one another, building a common curriculum and being involved in shared research processes augurs well for the profession. All countries have a very real role to play in promoting and indeed advocating health care as we approach the third millennium. Student and tutor exchanges are already taking place on the international scene. The future will surely see a free-flowing migration of both tutors and students between international institutions of higher education working on common subject areas and carrying the credit for work undertaken abroad back home to their mother institution where the work may be accredited as if the work had been undertaken at the mother institution. This will become the norm for students rather than the exception and will prove to be beneficial for all concerned.

The fine-tuning strategy that Gibbs has referred to in his approach to improving the quality of student learning is perhaps the final element missing from the overall picture of delivering training. Fine-tuning iŝreally an ongoing process that should never stop. As educationalists we can never submit to the temptation that we have 'always got it right'. There should always be room for improvement, growth and development, and not only from the side of the student; the lecturer too has to develop. It is only when the lecturer or tutor has been through the process him or herself that he or she can actually see its beneficial stance within education and help students to traverse the same path themselves, and at the same time allow their work to contribute to the learning experience.

The fine-tuning is achieved by:

- allowing students to have a say in their destiny;
- allowing them the availability of negotiation within the framework of their chosen course;
- giving them the opportunity to utilize their own experiences and relate them to the course;
- giving them the opportunity to criticize themselves within a shared group format or peer group environment;
- allowing students the opportunity to grapple with knowledge in an active manner rather than becoming purely passive observers;
- creating an assessment environment in which constructive criticism can be raised and by which the student can go on to grow and develop and achieve higher standards;
- exposing the students to a wide variety of learning resources, including appropriate use of library facilities, competent use of appropriate audiovisual aids (AVA), access to computing and video suites.

As Gibbs rightly questions, 'How do students get access to the subject content in a way which involves active rather than passive learning?' (Gibbs, 1992). If we apply the term fine-tuning to a car we anticipate that afterwards the engine will run smoothly and efficiently. In much the same way, in delivering training, the lecturer hopes that the student will find the path of education a smooth and efficient one. Being aware of the possibilities of what can be done within the educational setting and being responsive and open to possibilities of change and negotiation from students the lecturer can provide an experience which it is hoped will be an enriching one for both parties concerned.

ASSESSMENT, COMPETENCY AND UPDATING

The assessment of the capabilities of students is currently largely twofold:

1. through the use of continuous assessments in both common core areas and within the specialism of OH principles and practice;
2. through reports from fieldwork supervisors that are used to help to augment the overall profile of the student.

The assessment procedure normally requires the student to produce an assignment of approximately 3000 words in length following all the normal protocols for submission of an academic piece of work, in terms of content, style, referencing and bibliography. Assignments are normally typewritten or word-processed in the computer suite to produce good quality scripts. The work is given a deadline for submission to the marking tutor. A mark above 40% is regarded as a pass; anything below is referred for further submission but can then only score a maximum of 40% on resubmission if the examiners feel the piece of work is now acceptable for a pass grade, irrespective of how well the assignment may have been written. This is in fairness to those students who were successful on their first submission. Candidates need to have attended the university for a minimum of 80% of the time. Placement experience carries a requirement of a 100% attendance rate, as this piece of academic experience is crucial to the assignments undertaken within the specialism of OH.

Fieldwork supervisors' (FWS) reports obtained from placement experiences are a useful guide to both student and tutor to see if the theory that has been gained is being put into practice with useful effect. The report is a useful tool and means of assessing practical and practice based work. The report is normally written in conjunction with the student and the student has full knowledge of what the report contains. When the student returns to the university both student and tutor can take the opportunity to discuss the report through formal tutorial sessions. The FWSs occupy a unique position within the educational team as they have the opportunity to see students working directly with clients. They also have the experience and knowledge of students' work with other professionals/colleagues which is a vital part of the working role of a nurse regardless of specialism. The FWS report is a useful tool for identifying objectives for the future. It highlights areas which can be worked on even when the course is finished.

In the main the FWS report is concentrated around four key areas:

- Personality
- Interaction
- Knowledge
- Professionalism.

Whether they are being assessed by an FWS or the assignment tutor it is of great importance that students receive appropriate and constructive feedback as soon as possible, so that the learning experience can be enriched. Feedback which is delayed or unconstructive is a complete waste of time and serves no useful purpose for either the giver or receiver. Within the educational setting we hear more and more about National Vocational Qualifications (NVQs) and competency levels which NVQs are alleged to measure. Thomas (1992) states that 'if government targets are to be met, there will be no less than 12 million people – one half of the British workforce – pursuing NVQs by 1996'. Yet OHNs still seem to be in the dark about them and wonder if they have any reason to be concerned about them, or indeed what they are in the first place, and why the government has placed so much importance on them.

NVQs originated from a review undertaken of our skilled workforce in the early 1980s and comparative studies undertaken with our European competitors. The results showed that England and Wales were far behind other countries when it came to training people with the skills needed for the occupations they were to be employed in. The aim then was to redress the balance as quickly as possible and raise the profile of vocational training nationwide. Vocational qualifications were defined by Fletcher (1992) as: 'A statement of competence, clearly relevant to work and intended to facilitate entry into or progression in employment, further education and training, issued by a recognised body to an individual'. Therefore NVQs and their achievement imply that the skills of those who are awarded such qualifications are based on standards of competence set by a Lead Body and that they may be considered competent to undertake the task demanded of them. Competence then is a term that has become synonymous with NVQs. In order to find out what the competencies are for a specific job, the National Council for Vocational Qualifications (NCVQ) turn to the people who are considered the professionals in the area to be tested. The consultation process goes on with more and more bodies being asked to discuss and draw up information relating to a wide variety of occupations and to formulate competencies for such occupations that can be measured and assessed.

Competencies have already been written for people working in the health care field, e.g. ambulance personnel. In 1990 the Occupational Health and Safety Lead Body (OHSLB) was established to draw up competency standards for occupational health and safety practitioners. One of the chief criticisms about the OHSLB is that it has neglected to fully inform one of the very groups of people that NVQs in this field would affect, i.e. the OHN. A group of nurses in a variety of fields including OH and education, managers and OH consultants have formed an advisory group known as OHNTAG (the Occupational

Health Nursing Technical Advisory Group) which is raising important issues with the UKCC and NCVQ and trying to make sure that the NVQs, if they are to be inevitable for the profession, are created and adapted by OH nursing professionals and not by employers who so often in the past have set the competency standards for their own NVQs.

A recent study undertaken by the Health and Safety Executive looked at managers' perceptions of the role of the OHN. The study indicated that managers have a very poor perception of what OHNs are about. A review of the research in *The Newsletter* (1994) states, 'Lay managers see OHNs' role as a treatment service for injury or illness at work. The study shows that both doctor and lay managers showed little interest in management courses for OHNs'. Do OHNs wish them to be dictating what their tasks should be within their own specialism? As Bannister (1994) rightly asks, 'Who is leading whom? The clear emphasis of the NVQ approach is that industry leads and employers approve the qualification standards via the Lead Body; although there is a consultation phase with the professions, the qualification is quite clearly employer- and not profession-led'.

Over the next 12 months the debate will certainly increase in temperature in respect of competencies for OH nursing and many OHNs will surely have a voice which they will wish to have heard on the subject that affects them directly. It is quite possible that NVQs may have a very real place in the future of nurse education especially within task orientated skills procedures. NVQs might actually enhance the practice that OHNs undertake. They could create a very true and measurable outcome that quantifies a person's aptitude and competence for the role to be undertaken. Whatever the outcome the debate continues, but within the debate those involved in the task should make sure that OHNs are seen as driving the debate and not simply being passengers within the proceedings.

Bannister (1994) gives several requirements in relation to NVQs saying: 'NVQ may be a very good route to follow but it has to mature and grow before professional groups feel comfortable with its direction and concepts . . . What is required is for the profession to shout for what they want for the future of nurse education'.

These then are very interesting times. On the one hand we have tremendous opportunities developing within the traditional field of higher education relating to occupational health. OHNs can now obtain their DipHE and go on to take a higher degree qualification. There are opportunities to undertake Masters degrees in practitioner research and on to PhD. At the same time, on the other hand, a debate continues which might radically change the way in which qualifications are obtained. The debate on NVQs will run for quite some time but it is doubtful that it will go away. As interested individuals within the specialism of OH, OHNs have to be more than just bystanders but need to take an active part in discussion and debate on such issues that may shape the future of professional OH education.

It is possible that NVQs may have even more relevance and a more important role to play within the Post Registration Education and Practice Project (PREPP). Continuous updating might lend itself more easily to the NVQ approach of obtaining units of accreditation. Furthermore, the UKCC's recently published strategy for implementation of PREPP would seem to be trying to enable nurses to have the opportunity to achieve their five days study leave every three years through a 'variety of activities'. Could this mean NVQ style units that nurses, including OHNs, could tap into? Fortunately for many OHNs who might find it difficult to obtain time off from their employment it would seem that the UKCC's criteria may be satisfied and achieved by undertaking study activities within practice and therefore not having to take time out of work. There are many ways in which personal development and portfolio enhancement can be developed after registration and the DipHE course should provide OHNs with the tools to undertake activities such as: risk and hazard assessment; investigating new approaches to care; the treatment of patients; undertaking personal research and the publication of results; analysis of patient support which might include such skills as counselling strategies and techniques; and auditing the service to make it run more efficiently for both employee, employer and OHN.

The ENB has stated in its dealings with the professional portfolio that all practice-based nurses, which should include OHNs, need to focus their professional development on maintaining and improving the quality of care they provide for patients and clients. Continuous updating is part and parcel of such development. It should be welcomed wholeheartedly by all who care about their profession and those who would be called 'professional' and those who care about the specialism of OH. Gone are the days when OHNs, or any other specialism for that matter, could think that once they had been appointed they could sit back and wait for retirement to come. The OHN of today has to be aware that OH is a continuously developing service and that the service dies without practitioners who continue to look at areas that can be improved and elaborated on to bring out the optimum type of service for both clients and the profession.

Clearly the OHN of today has to be both professional and managerial, but also educational in all aspects of his/her work. The OHN has by necessity to educate not only employees but managers, employers and all whom the specialism comes into contact with. If non-nursing professionals have a poor idea or understanding of what the OHN role is about it's up to the OHN to redress the balance and make him or herself accountable by showing what exactly can be done, displaying the cost benefits of proposed undertakings and above all by making sure that people understand that nursing in occupational health is not a myth but very much a real need. As educationalists we have to meet the needs of our clients whether we look at the term 'clients' to mean 'students' or 'prospective employers'. We need to make sure that our students are prepared for the 'real' world of occupational health so that they can work as equals in a positive way in order to achieve and set their own goals.

The words of Stachtchenko and Janicek (1990), although not aimed at the OHN, are nevertheless relevant: 'During the past few years the concept of health has taken on a more dynamic connotation and now includes the ability of individuals to respond positively to their environments and thus achieve their potential'. It is clear that the OHN of today and the OHN of the third millennium will need by necessity to be 'streetwise' in relation to the multifactorial influences that may impinge on the role. The OHN will have to speak the language of economist, manager, politician, environmentalist, to mention but a few. The OHN cannot afford to shelter within the confines of a simple health care model, passive and unresponsive. Much will be demanded of this ever developing and changing role and the OHN today must prepare for the demands of tomorrow. As educationalists we must reflect on this and aim to reach the goal of achieving a quality product that serves the needs of industry, today, tomorrow and into the future.

REFERENCES

Alston, R. *et al.* (1988) The Hanasaari conceptual model for occupational health nursing. Paper presented at the RCN OHN Forum, Subland.

Bannister, C. (1994) To lead or to follow? Dilemma of the NVQ. *Occupational Health Journal*, **46**(1), 12–16.

Brown, L.R., *et al.* (1993) *State of the World 1993*, Earthscan Publications Ltd, London, UK.

Fairburn, J. and McGettigan, J. (1994) Development of an OH Management model: part 1. *Occupational Health Journal*, **46**(4), 120–23.

Fletcher, S. (1992) *NVQs, Standards and Competence*, Kogan Page, London, UK.

Garvey, J.P. (1993a) As educationalists are we meeting the needs of industry today? Huddersfield University, MEd Assignment into Issues and Problem Analysis (unpublished).

Garvey, J.P. (1993b) Learning to study the independent way. *Occupational Health Journal*, **45**(6), 206–8.

Garvey, J.P. (1994) Nursing in Occupational Health, Myth or Realistic Need? Huddersfield University, MEd Assignment into Research Methods (unpublished).

Gibbs, G. (1992) *Improving the Quality of Student Learning.* Technical and Educational Services Ltd, Bristol, UK.

Hodgkinson, M. (1992) *A Higher Education Credit Accumulation and Transfer Strategy for Europe*, HMSO, London, UK.

The Newsletter of the Royal College of Nursing, Society of Occupational Health Nursing (1994) Winter Issue, London, UK, p. 11.

Schon, D.A. (1983) *The Reflective Practitioner*, Temple Smith, London, UK.

Schon, D.A. (1987) *Educating the Reflective Practitioner*, Jossey-Bass, San Francisco, USA.

Stachtchenko, S. and Janicek, M. (1990) Conceptual differences between prevention and health promotion: research implications for community health programs. *Canadian Journal of Public Health*, **81**, 53–9.

Thomas, H. (1992) All about NVQs. *Progress Journal*, September, 25–6.

PART FOUR

Information sources and services   12

Sheila Pantry

Information is vital in today's society; it is needed in every walk of life but none more than in the OSH field. For the manager this will mean acquiring up-to-date knowledge of the legislation including the European directives, the various interpretations, guidance, advice, and research results.

There are exciting trends and developments in OSH information provision. No longer does the organization need to aim to collect every document just in case it needs to refer to it. It is more a question of 'just-in-time' delivery as these systems and services develop and become even more user friendly.

Since the Robens report was issued, the last two decades have seen the delivery of information become computerized alongside software packages being developed to meet the needs of businesses both large and small.

What does all this mean for those who wish to be a successful OSH manager?

In today's technology based industries and processes questions are being asked by increasingly knowledgeable workforces who will need the answer if not 'on the spot' then fairly quickly after asking it! Therefore, given that it is not necessary to automatically acquire every piece of information, to be a successful OSH manager in the 1990s will require a wide appreciation of a number of skills and abilities, one of which will be the ability to obtain up-to-date information which has been validated and is authoritative. The need to be able to obtain information via the computer will be paramount. The OSH manager will need to acquire a personal computer which will assist in a number of ways to make the work flow more cost effectively:

- in planning health and safety audits for the organization;
- keeping statistics and records of accidents, injuries and ill health;

- writing health and safety manual and instructions;
- keeping records of inspection reviews of plant and machinery as required by legislation;
- accessing compact discs read-only memory (CD-ROMs).

Even in these days of deregulation the OSH manager has to keep up to date as revision and updating of the legislation takes place alongside new legislation. Most of the OSH legislation is coming from the European Union and is based on the concept of risk assessment. If the organization does not have a competent person to carry out the assessment then one may need to be found. 'May' is a very important word, because this is where information becomes even more important to the OSH manager. Many authoritative and validated publications abound and knowledge of their existence and contents could save time and money when seeking solutions to workplace problems. So the wise OSH manager will find the information first before any outside help is called in.

What is information and where to find it? Everyone believes that they know the answer to this question, but the following may expand the knowledge base of OSH managers and others seeking up-to-date information.

LEGISLATION

As OSH legislation mostly emanates from Europe, the OSH information seeker will need to be aware that details of new proposals, amendments, directives, recommendations, etc. will be published in the European Union's *Official Journal*. Note that this has two main series – the 'L' series and the 'C' series. It is worth checking the *Official Journal* for early warning of impending new UK legislation.

As these new pieces of European legislation are adopted in the UK, legislation details will be found in press releases from the Health and Safety Executive/Commission. These press releases can be acquired on a subscription basis from HSE Books, PO Box 1999, Sudbury, Suffolk CO10 6FS, UK, Tel: +44 (0)1787 881165 or Fax: +44 (0)1787 313995 for details. A new subscription service which provides information about HSE publications started in April 1994. Journals and newsletters all thrive on the HSC/E press releases so these will no doubt pick up all the details of any new legislation. It is important to watch the developments in the **deregulation arena** – 1994/95 will produce some interesting results for those working in occupational safety and health.

Her Majesty's Stationery Office (HMSO) is still responsible for printing and selling copies of legislation so apply to HMSO for a standing order. The latest (second) edition of *Redgrave, Fife and Machin on Health and Safety* published by Butterworths at the end of 1993, will give the reader an overview of the current state of play. This volume will be updated by an annual supplement.

For an overview from the European Union point of view *The European Communities' Health and Safety Legislation* by Frank Wright and Alan Neal, published by Chapman & Hall, gives details of the new directives, etc. A second volume to update the first will be available later in 1995; likewise a volume on chemical safety legislation will be produced by the same authors.

GUIDES TO HEALTH AND SAFETY AT WORK LEGISLATION IN THE UK

A number of publications in addition to those mentioned above which will assist in understanding the implications of the law on health and safety at work are briefly described below.

CRONER'S HEALTH AND SAFETY AT WORK

This is produced as a loose-leaf book with bimonthly updates and is intended to be used as a guide to the content and location of detailed legal safety requirements. Acts of Parliament are paraphrased but judicial interpretations are not usually incorporated. The book seeks to be comprehensive in that it attempts to include some reference to every regulatory control which relates to the reduction of hazards associated with work activity, but it is selective in that it has placed more emphasis on those controls which in the view of the editors have most significance for subscribers to a reference book of this nature. It explains how the UK system of regulation operates and has a very extensive key word index so that the reader is referred exactly to the subject. There is also a brief description of the state of legislation. After purchase there is an annual charge for the amendment service.

CRONER'S REFERENCE BOOK FOR EMPLOYERS

Again a loose-leaf book with monthly updates, it provides accurate, clear information on the whole range of legislative provisions on health and safety at work, in addition to comprehensive coverage of most aspects of employment legislation. It is not intended primarily for the OHS practitioner but it contains enough on the subject to be useful if *Redgrave's Health and Safety in Factories* is not available. It is now available on floppy disk.

CRONER'S HEALTH AND SAFETY CASE LAW

A loose-leaf format with quarterly updates which aims to clarify the grey areas in the wide ranging health and safety legislation, by bringing together cases which have been through the courts and the judgments of which could be influential on future cases.

CRONER'S ENVIRONMENT MANAGEMENT

Loose-leaf format with quarterly updates, which covers the full implications of environmental protection, detailing relevant legislation, the UK situation and the administratrative arrangements in the UK and the European Union.

OTHER PUBLICATIONS

Health and Safety at Work Handbook by M.A. Dewis edited by J. Braune is published by Tolley Publishing Co. The latest edition includes changes in the legislation.

Encyclopaedia of health and safety at work: law and practice published by Sweet & Maxwell offers authoritative guidance on the fast moving health and safety legislation. In three volumes, the encyclopaedia gives the full text of the relevant pieces of legislation. The subscription includes an updating service for the year of purchase. An excellent source of reliable information.

A Guide to the Health and Safety at Work etc. Act 1974 (4th edn) is published by HSE Books and is the HSE definitive guide to the Act.

The HSE Information Service issues two lists which are designed to assist the information seeker. Both are free of charge from the HSE Information Centre, Broad Lane, Sheffield S3 7HQ UK, Tel: +44 (0)1142 892345, Fax: +44 (0)1142 892333. The lists are as follows:

• Legislation pre and post the Health and Safety at Work etc. Act.
• Forms used in conjunction with legislation.

Both lists are lengthy, comprehensive and very informative.

For Online and CD-ROM legal information see pp. 290–6.

OPEN LEARNING COURSES AND LEGISLATION

As new legislation is issued a number of successful open learning packages have been developed by the Health and Safety Executive to help the OSH manager to acquire knowledge in a step-by-step approach. A good example in the health area is on the Control of Substances Hazardous to Health Regulations (COSHH).

JOURNALS

OSH-type journals are published by institutional or commercial publishers and carry articles on topical subjects, a diary of events, and many others pieces of information on new publications, systems, services, products and commentary. The OSH manager may need to take more than one journal in order to be informed and also be on the mailing list for any new information coming out from the publishers, institutions, government organizations, etc.

To be able to obtain information appearing in back issues of journals the information seeker needs to be able to locate libraries and information services holding these titles. Consequently, a need for a list of such titles with locations was recognized and has been compiled by the UK Occupational Safety and Health Information Group (OSHIG), entitled *What's Where* (available from Dr M. Hannant, Royal Society of Chemistry, Thomas Graham House, Science Park, Milton Road, Cambridge CB4 4WF, Tel: +44 (0)1223 420066, Fax: +44 (0)1223 423429). Because there are increasing difficulties in the UK in being able to locate libraries and information services holding OSH journals who would be willing to provide photocopies or loan the journal, this list is invaluable. It locates journals that are available from organizations willing to help.

Currently, the most common vehicle for information is paper, in the form of books and periodical publications. These periodicals appear on a regular schedule, and the books have extensive, well-established distribution networks. The 'primary literature' is the set of journals where new observations, discoveries or inventions are reported by the people responsible. State-of-the-art reviews also appear in primary publications. To be published in a primary publication, an article must be reviewed by a number of experts in the given field, who will ensure that it reflects good practice and that its conclusions follow from the facts presented.

This process is called 'peer review'. Examples are the *American Industrial Hygiene Association Journal*, *Journal of Occupational Medicine*, *Occupational and Environmental Medicine* (formerly *British Journal of Industrial Medicine*), *Scandinavian Journal of Work, Environment and Health*, and *Ergonomics*.

Typical of the 'other' category are *Occupational Health*, and the *Journal of the American Medical Association* (*JAMA*) and other medical journals. Primary journals can be found in the libraries of appropriate institutions (*JAMA* in medical school and hospital libraries, for example).

There are some core mass circulation magazines that are not peer reviewed, but do provide primary information in the form of news of recent or upcoming events, in addition to easy-to-read articles on topics of current interest. They often include advertisements for OSH products and services that are themselves useful information on sources of supply. They may be published by public authorities, e.g. the *Health and Safety Commission Newsletter* or by private publishers or institutions/ societies, e.g. *Safety Management* (British Safety Council), *Health and Safety at Work* (Tolley), *Occupational Safety and Health* (RoSPA), *Safety and Health Practitioner* (IOSH). There are many publications directed toward other specialities that include useful or interesting information: *Chemical Week*, *Plant Engineer*, *Fire Prevention*.

SECONDARY SOURCES

The difficulty in finding information on one particular topic in the mass of the primary literature has prompted the development of 'secondary sources'. These are guides to the literature or to recent events, such as court cases, whose official write-ups appear elsewhere. They tell where a given document on a particular topic was published and usually give a brief summary of its contents. There are also 'citation indexes', which list the publications that have cited a given document; these permit very efficient retrieval of relevant publications once one key reference has been identified (unfortunately, there is none devoted exclusively to OSH). Because they must be completely up-to-date, secondary sources use the latest electronic technology to speed their publication. In fact most are offered in electronic form as well as in print. Some core titles are: *Safety and Health at Work*, ILO-CIS Bulletin; Excerpta Medica *Occupational Health and Industrial Medicine*; CA selects *Occupational Safety and Health*. Others are: *Science Citation Index*, *Social Science Citation Index*, *Chemical Abstracts*, *BIOSIS*. Because of the number of highly trained people involved in their preparation, secondary sources tend to be expensive.

Some updating services, e.g. Croners, Sweet & Maxwell, are valuable secondary sources as they cite important recent publications, laws or court decisions. Whereas many government publications of the type are free, the privately researched and compiled newsletters tend to be expensive. They are rare in libraries; those who need them find them worth the price of subscription.

OTHER SOURCES

A third major type of information source includes textbooks, encyclopaedias and compendia. Whereas reviews in the primary literature describe a domain of knowledge at the time of writing, tertiary-source reviews recount the evolution of that knowledge and its larger context.

Compendia of data bring together values originally measured and reported at different times over many years.

Useful textbooks for the OSH information seeker can be found listed in guides and sources (Pantry, 1992) and Cherrie and McGovern (1993). In these guides are listed well-known books such as *Patty's Industrial Hygiene and Toxicology; Ridley's Safety at Work; Harrington and Gill's Occupational Health; Sax's Dangerous Properties of Industrial Materials;* and *Casarett and Doull's Toxicology*. In addition the guides, which cost together £20, give other sources of information listed under various headings which will direct the information seeker quickly to validated and authoritative information.

ORGANIZATIONS

Perhaps the range of organizations issuing OSH information is not known to everyone, particularly those newly entering the field. Government departments and agencies such as the Health and Safety Executive, the Department of Health and the Department of Trade and Industry are prime producers of OSH information. Other organizations on an international or European level will also be valuable sources of OSH information. Major producers are the International Labour Office in Geneva, the World Health Organization, the International Social Security Association, the European Foundation for Living and Working Conditions. They all issue a wide range of publications written by experts.

Membership of organizations such as the British Occupational Hygiene Society, the British Safety Council, the Fire Protection Association, the Institution of Occupational Safety and Health, the Royal College of Nursing, the Royal Society for the Prevention of Accidents, the Society of Occupational Medicine, to name a few, would be of use. Membership would be one way of keeping up to date and also having access to others working in the field. Likewise it is useful to belong to local OSH groups which act as networks and enable members to exchange information on current issues.

Other handbooks/yearbooks will list organizations; examples are the *Croner's Health and Safety Directory at Work;* the *EHAS Group Environmental Health and Safety Yearbook, Health and Safety Manager's Yearbook* by AP Information Services and ROSPA.

The Health and Safety Executive Information Services issues a free list entitled *Organizations concerned with health and safety information*. It gives details of organizations, addresses, telephone and fax numbers, contact person, status of organization, principle functions and activities. A useful reference source for the busy OSH manager and information seeker!

STANDARD SPECIFICATIONS

Very important sources of OHS information which cannot be ignored are Standard Specifications. Some years ago the UK government expressed a determination to enhance the status of standards and quality assurance with the object of increasing industrial efficiency, including safety, and strengthening international competitiveness by issuing a White Paper by the Department of Trade entitled *Standards, Quality and International Competitiveness*, HMSO, 1982, Cmnd 8621, ISBN 0101862505. In addition, the European Union has also promulgated a policy of harmonization of standard specifications in a wide area of work activities.

Most countries have a standardization body which prepares, organizes and promulgates national standards. Usually the national standardization body is represented on international bodies for standardization, thus ensuring harmonization and cooperation of action. The scope of standards work includes glossaries of terms, definitions, quantities, units and symbols, methods of testing, preferred signs and styles, codes of practice and safety, health and environment requirements.

The Health and Safety Commission (HSC) in the *Plan of Work 1985–86 and Onwards* stated: 'Standard making is regarded as an economical and effective route to safety and health and intends to continue to make a major contribution to the development of the British Standards System'.

Risk assessment can contribute to successful management of health and safety and the OSH manager will need to be aware of the many standards, particularly British Standards, which set good and achievable standards in tasks carried out in the workplace. Many of the British Standards have been written in collaboration with the Health and Safety Executive. To encourage firms to know what is expected of them and their competitors and to promote greater use of British Standards, the Health and Safety Executive has identified over 1400 Standards which are significant to health and safety at work. Many British Standards are cited in the HSC/E publications as well as listed in the OSH-CD (see pp. 292–5).

Standardization bodies such as the British Standards Institution are also concerned with certification and assessment of products and with the international aspects of the subject. The usual principles observed in the preparation of standards are that they should be in accordance with the needs of the economy, should meet a generally recognized demand and take into account the interest of producers and users. Standards are usually prepared under the guidance of representative committees and are widely circulated before they are authorized for publication. They are normally listed in a yearbook, catalogue or database.

Occasionally the standardization body will issue a collection of standards on a subject, e.g. a list of standards on safety equipment. Most catalogues or yearbooks will have a subject to help the user. Databases will also retrieve standards by subject.

BSI has a number of addresses as follows: Head Office, 389 Chiswick High Road London W4 4BL, Tel: +44 (0)181 996 9000, Fax: +44 (0)181 996 7400; also at Linford Wood, Milton Keynes, MK14 6LE. For subscriptions and other enquiries telephone +44 (0)1908 220022.

HOW TO FIND BRITISH STANDARDS

BSI publishes an annual catalogue which is as up-to-date as possible and lists all British Standard Specifications (BSS) in numerical order – the general list first and then the various series. Each entry gives the number, part number, year of publication, title, size, amendments issued, technical committee references, certification marking and any corresponding international standards. There is also a brief abstract describing the contents of the Standard. Towards the end of the catalogue there is a useful numerical list of international standards corresponding to the British Standards. An alphabetical subject index is also included. The indexing of the Standards has improved over the years but could be improved still further, so when searching for an item persist in thinking of alternative terms to find the subject of the standard needed and do not just look, for example, under the term 'safety'.

The BSI catalogue is updated by the *BSI Catalogue Supplement* which is a cumulative publication, issued monthly, and is available on subscription to members of BSI. It lists for the period since the compilation of the catalogue all new and revised publications, amendments, items withdrawn and European Standards issued. For details of subscriptions contact BSI. *BSI News*, a monthly publication which announces new Standards, withdrawals, revisions, and amendments, also includes articles and news items. It should also be noted that complete sets of British Standards are maintained in some, but not all, major towns and cities in public and other libraries. Check with BSI for details of the locations. Some overseas countries also hold complete sets of British Standards Specifications (BSS) in various locations such as the national standardization body.

BRITISH STANDARDS INSTITUTION LIBRARY LOANS

The BSI library holds about half a million foreign and international standards, codes of practice, regulations and technical requirements.

Most of these are available for loan to UK subscribing members of BSI in exchange for library tokens which can be purchased from the BSI sales department. BSI publications are not available for loan. Requests to borrow documents can be made by telephone, fax or letter.

STANDARDS JOURNALS

Current journals issued by the various standards bodies can also be referred to, together with material about standards theory and practice. Overseas and international standards, some of which have been translated into English, may be borrowed by subscribing members of BSI. Full particulars from Subscriptions Department at Milton Keynes.

PLUS

BSI recognizes that as standards are subject to constant change, maintaining an up-to-date collection is not easy. PLUS (Private Line Updating Service) takes care of this task for you. Simply send BSI your list of Standards. Any collection of standards can be updated – British, international, foreign/national – and they will validate the list and send you a monthly report on any revisions or changes. The service includes the automatic supply of updated standards and if you operate a quality system, a twice yearly audit list can also be supplied. Contact BSI Sales for further details. For details of computerized services see pp. 290–6.

FILMS AND VIDEOS

Films and videos are an important way of highlighting accidents and malpractices in the working environment. A number of organizations in the UK produce films and videos on a regular basis. Many 'Open Learning' courses use videos as one of the training aids. Health and safety magazines review and list new films and videos.

The following have been selected from the range of films and videos available. The full range of suppliers of audiovisual material is far too long to list, but there are general catalogues which jointly give a fuller coverage. Most catalogues are free of charge.

The British Film Institute, 21 Dean St, London W1P 1PL, Tel: +44 (0)171 255 1444, Fax: +44 (0)171 436 7950 produces a catalogue four times per year entitled *British Film and Video Catalogue*, which is a subject listing of recent material on management and related topics. Under Health and Safety the listing covers a broad range of subjects. Details are given of where to hire or buy films and videos, and includes a list of distributors' and production companies' names and addresses.

The British Medical Association, BMA House, Tavistock Square,

London WC1H 9JP, Tel: +44 (0)171 387 4499, Fax: +44 (0)171 388 2544, have a Film and Video service which stocks one of the largest collections of medical and health material in Europe.

The British Safety Council, National Safety Centre, Chancellors Rd, London W6 9RS, Tel: +44 (0)181 741 1231/2371, Fax: +44 (0)181 741 0835/4555 produces a guide which includes films, videos and tape/slide presentations. The sections in the guide include accident prevention, hazard control, supervision and management, eye safety, noise, fire, fork lift trucks and hospital safety. There is also a section which advises where you can obtain the equipment to show the material. The BSC monthly magazine *Safety Management* lists new films, videos, etc. as they are issued.

CFL Vision, PO Box 35, Wetherby, West Yorkshire, LS23 7EX, Tel: +44 (0)1937 541010, Fax: +44 (0)1937 541083, is part of the Central Office of Information, and stocks many hundreds of titles on 16 mm film and video cassettes, available on hire (sometimes free) and for sale. Contact CFL for a copy of its catalogue. HSC/E films and videos are available from CFL Vision.

The Health and Safety Executive has produced over 30 films and videos since 1975. The films/videos, on a variety of subjects, are available for hire or purchase from CFL Vision (see above for address, etc). HSE Information Services also produces annually an extensive catalogue called *Audio visual resources in health and safety: films, videos and tape slide material available from distributors in the UK*. Contact HSE Public Enquiry Point, Tel: +44 (0)1142 892345, Fax: +44 (0)1142 892333 for details of current catalogue and price.

The Royal Society for the Prevention of Accidents, Cannon House, The Priory, Queensway, Birmingham B9 6BS, Tel: +44 (0)121 200 2461, Fax: +44 (0)121 200 1254. Video Review, a feature appearing regularly in RoSPA's magazine *Occupational Safety and Health* cites new products and gives an appraisal as well as price for hire or purchase. There is also a RoSPA Film/Video Library catalogue.

Videotel Marine International Ltd, Ramillies House, 1/2 Ramillies St, London W1V 1DF, Tel: +44 (0)171 439 6301, Fax: +44 (0)171 437 0731, Telex: 298596, produces and distributes safety and technical training films as 16 mm films and video cassettes in most languages, and sold internationally through their own offices and agents. Originally aimed at the shipping industry, it now produces packages covering a whole range of topics, e.g. catering, offshore oil, first aid.

MICROFICHE

Barbour has been set up to provide vital reference information for safety officers, representatives, inspectors and all others responsible for complying with or administrating the Health and Safety at Work etc. Act 1974. The microfile is reproduced on microfiche and contains the full text of publications ranging from legislation to standards and codes, advisory leaflets and data sheets, from a host of suppliers – some large, some small, ranging from the British Standards Institution, the Department of Health, the Fire Research Station, and the Health and Safety Executive to the Royal College of Nursing.

The microfile has a number of sub-sets which can be purchased together or separately. The subject range is expanding: as well as health and safety, there are sets on Environmental Health Services; Fire Safety and Security Services; European Supplement; Offshore and Maritime Safety; and Eire supplement. The microfile is updated, expanded and a new index published three times per year. If no information facilities exist in an organization, then this is one way of ensuring that all essential documents from selected authoritative sources are immediately available. Barbour continue to expand its microfile services, details of which are available from Barbour Index plc, New Lodge, Drift Rd, Windsor, Berkshire S14 4RQ, Tel: +44 (0)1344 884121, Fax: +44 (0)1344 884845.

CHADWYCK-HEALEY

Another useful service started in 1980 is the *Catalogue of British Official Publications not published by HMSO*, produced by Chadwyck-Healey Ltd, Cambridge, Tel: +44 (0)1223 215512, Fax: +44 (0)1223 215513. The catalogue, which is published monthly and cumulates annually, covers the publications of over 400 organizations financed or controlled completely by the UK government, which are not produced by HMSO. The Health and Safety Executive, Health Education Council and also the Department of Health are amongst the organizations whose publications are included and are available from Chadwyck-Healey on microfiche. Publications can be bought in five ways: as individual titles; as publications of individual publishing bodies; as subject collections (e.g. employment and working conditions would include health and safety at work); as major collections; or as the complete collection. A useful service, it ensures that an organization does not have to continually chase documents individually.

Chadwyck-Healey has collaborated with HMSO to produce a compact disc read-only memory (CD-ROM) known as UKOP. This product covers as comprehensively as possible all the health and safety related documents published both by HMSO and government departments and agencies.

ROLE OF TECHNOLOGY IN HEALTH AND SAFETY INFORMATION DISSEMINATION

WHAT KIND OF A COMPUTER?

Mainframe computers will handle a wide variety of jobs, but a personal computer (PC) will meet most OSH managers' and practitioners' requirements and can be bought for about £1200, printers from about £150 for a basic type to the more sophisticated laser printers costing from £700 upwards.

A compact disc drive (reader) can be obtained for about £300; note that some come more cheaply but are not able to read some of the CD-ROMs which are available in health and safety subjects. The following requirements are recommended if a variety of tasks including the use of compact discs is envisaged:

- 486 IBM compatible PC or Pentium range
- 8 MB or more of RAM (random access memory)
- 120 MB or larger hard disk
- MS-DOS or PC-DOS 5.0 or higher
- Expanded memory (EMS) emulator (memory manager)
- MS-DOS CD-ROM extensions 2.1 or higher
- ISO 9660 compatible CD-ROM drive
- VGA colour monitor
- one high density floppy drive (preferably two) 3.5″ and 5.25″
- one parallel port for a printer
- one mouse or pointer device.

WHAT KIND OF SOFTWARE?

PCs are versatile and there is a good selection of software available which can help the OSH manager in the following ways:

- Office procedures
  - writing letters/reports
  - producing safety manuals
  - keeping a diary/calendar of when audit checks need to be carried out
  - producing a mailing list.

Software such as AmiPro, Word, WordPerfect, and Wordstar will help the OSH manager

- Information retrieval
  - index information kept in the office by using software such as dBase III Plus or IV; Dataease; Foxpro

- access remote computers by contacting the online host services such as IRS/Dialtech, Datastar, Dialog, STN, National Chemical Emergency Centre, Harwell (which has other computerized services available for the PC user)
- use CD-ROMs; the software is supplied either with, or integrated within, the CD-ROM by suppliers such as SilverPlatter, CCOHS, Sigma Aldrich
- floppy disks and other services such as those offered by Buildings and Health supplied by H & H Scientific Consultants; SAFECHEM from Sergeant Safety Supplies
- Unique applications
  - keeping logs of accident and incident reports
  - risk assessments
  - keeping statistics
  - keeping records
  - stock control on equipment, fire extinguishers, materials (time limits and disposal times)
  - safety date sheets.

Services and systems such as CHAOSS supplied by ICL/General Research Corporation; COSHH Administration by Cognisoft; COSHH-DM by Corporate Management Services (BNFL); FLOW GEMINI from General Research Corp.; MicroCOSHH, MICROSAFE iii and MICROTRACK from Bowring Marsh and McLennan.

As these applications are installed on the computer the work flow will alter and become more organized but remember that it takes time to draw up a specification of a computer requirement and acquire and learn how to use all the facilities competently.

COMPUTERIZED OCCUPATIONAL HEALTH AND SAFETY INFORMATION

OHS information seekers should be aware that many of the printed paper versions of documents, catalogues, indexes and abstracts to the literature are also available on computers throughout the world. It is not now necessary to spend many hours travelling to sources of information, checking manually through periodicals, etc. or, worse, not being able to access the information at all.

Today information services worldwide are greatly influenced by developments in computer and communications technologies. Early application of computers to information emphasized organizing and managing document collections. Information centres and libraries of all kinds used mainframe computers to organize, catalogue, index, record, search and retrieve their information holdings. These became known as bibliographic databases and often contain many thousands of references. Each reference includes title, author(s), keywords/abstracts, and bibliographic citation including publisher and date of publication. For example, OSH bibliographic databases are: CISDOC, from the CIS; HSELINE, the UK Health and Safety Executive's database on occupational health and safety information; CCINFO, from the Canadian Centre for Occupational Health and Safety; NIOSHTICS, from the US National Institute of Occupational Safety and Health. There are also databases which have the full text of the documents rather than an abstract, e.g. LEXIS, which contains the full text of legal documents.

Another type of database comprises primarily numeric data. These are sometimes known as databanks, e.g. CHEMBANK. A list of databases which provide information on occupational health and safety are listed elsewhere in this chapter. This list is not comprehensive; other OHS information specialists will no doubt have other sources. It should also be appreciated that lists rapidly become out of date as new sources become available. A word of warning – because many of the databases are extracting from the same source documents, it is inevitable that when searches are carried out on a number of host services there will be duplication of references retrieved.

The vast majority of the documents published on scientific and technical information have been written by scientists and specialists for use by their peer groups. Today all sectors of society are demanding this information – academic, scientific, medical, legal, technical, social, trade, and also the general public.

Effective searching involves not only subject knowledge, but extensive search and retrieval skills. Structured databases containing even more factual databases have evolved over the years and through improvements in telecommunications systems and software systems have become accessible to many people located in all parts of the world. However, once the refences have been retrieved then the documents need to be obtained through a document delivery service or information service.

ONLINE SERVICES

Commercially available online services have proliferated during the last two decades, thus making information more easily accessible. At the end of 1994 there were estimated to be well over 6000 databases available for information retrieval in the world, covering many subjects and totalling over 100 million references. In addition there are over 2200 CD-ROM sources, including an ever increasing number of full text CD-ROMs.

Online services, which started with bibliographic databases, relied on huge central mainframe computers which are costly to establish and maintain. As the volume of information and the user population grow, the upgrading of the systems alone involves heavy investments.

'Open systems' which allow computers to talk to computers anywhere in the world are becoming part of the workplace environment, thus it is no longer necessary to host all the data needed on an 'in-house' computer.

Guides to online searching

There are a number of useful guides to online searching and databases which the OHS information seeker may wish to consult. Either contact the nearest public or university library and information service or they may be purchased from the publisher.

What is a database host?

A database host is an organization offering one or more databases/databanks on its mainframe computer for access by the public. These services are usually available round the clock, except for two to three hours in the very early morning in some cases. Some hosts offer databases on all subjects, some specialize in one subject area and some seek to have 'unique' databases, e.g. available only on their own computer system. These hosts will supply useful, easy to read booklets giving information for those beginning to work or thinking of working with online services for the first time. They assume no previous experience and give definitions of terminology, costs involved, contacts for help and details of further reading on all aspects of online searching.

How do online services work?

Access to online services is usually made from a visual display unit (VDU) and a teletype compatible terminal, a communicating word processor, or a personal computer with telecommunications software. A telephone and a modem are also needed. The modem converts the audible telephone signals and inputs them to the computer and reverses the process with signals output from the computer. All host services will give information on the equipment needed and methods of access, and will also train would-be searchers. Many public libraries and information brokers will make searches for those who do not have facilities or who do not wish to learn how to search.

Through the online systems, users can have immediate access to current information from bibliographic and direct subject databases from anywhere in the world and with the improved technologies available for finding the required information do not now need such sophisticated skills as online databases demanded when they first became available. Finding, managing and organizing bibliographic information can be made easier by using software programs which are relatively cheap to buy and use. All the database host services will give information seekers details of these packages as well as of their services and the databases hosted on their computer.

WHAT IS A CD-ROM?

In the 1980s the development of personal computers coupled with advances in 'compact disc read-only memory' (CD-ROM) technology brought about a revolution in the information world. It is now quite easy to have available vast amounts of information on a single $5\frac{1}{4}''$ or $3\frac{1}{2}''$ disc at a relatively low cost. Over 330 000 A4 sheets of information can be stored on one single disc. The information is read from the disc by a laser mounted in a special CD player which is linked to a personal computer. A printer will also be required if paper copies of the information are to be printed out. The computer should be IBM compatible, preferably with a 386 processor. A good monitor screen will be essential if users are going to spend long periods of time in front of the screen. The new European Union directive on display screens used for business purposes will need to be adhered to if employees are to have a satisfactory working environment. It is better to use screens which are 'enhanced graphics adapter' (EGA), 'multi colour graphics adapter' (MCGA) or 'video graphics adapter' (VGA).

Several features of CD-ROM make it an ideal vehicle for many users and many purposes. The costs of CD-ROMs, players and related hardware and software continue to drop, bringing them within the reach of almost every organization. Therefore the information is easily transportable and usable, thus enabling a huge amount of data to be stored and reused repeatedly without extra costs and reliance on intermediaries to find the information required. Users are also able to obtain it in the form that is best suited to their requirements. Sophisticated searchers and information users can take full advantage of databases and databanks of worldwide published and unpublished documents including journals. Direct subject databases on the various topics can be consulted for technical details or information for practical application. An example is the many databases on chemicals, their use, transportation regulations and disposal methods, etc. Such databases provide useful information to researchers and practitioners, as well as workplace technicians without a technical background, as do the range of full text CD-ROMs containing graphics/diagrams and pictures which may include poster-like summaries or instructions, or brief summary documents with images, or descriptions of practical applications.

NETWORKING CD-ROMS

When CD-ROMs were first produced, they were aimed at the single user of information using a personal computer. However, as technology has developed, software is now available which allows one or more CD-ROMs to be accessed across almost any PC network. The foundation of such a network is called a 'local area network' which connects a number of PC workstations together. The actual PC workstations can be located in a number of different rooms. The network software is loaded onto one PC which acts as a 'file server' or 'network server'. A variety of network software packages are available.

The following will give the OSH manager details of the contents of various OSH related CD-ROMs.

OSH-ROM will give access to four major databases containing references to worldwide sources of information. The databases are:

- NIOSHTIC, from the United States National Institute of Occupational Safety and Health (NIOSH). The database contains valuable references to all NIOSH documents such as Criteria Documents, Occupational Hazard Assessments, Special Hazard Reviews, Joint Occupational Health Recommendations, Current Intelligence Bulletins, Manual of Analytical Methods, also references to journals, reports, books and other documents mainly from the USA.
- CISDOC from the International Labour Office Health and Safety Centre, Geneva covers references from many countries which are linked into the Centre. The coverage includes legislation, research results, material and chemical safety data sheets, conference proceedings and journal articles.
- MHIDAS from AEA Technology Ltd, UK gives detailed summaries of the chemical industry accidents and incidents showing the loss of life and the extent of the accidents.
- HSELINE, the Health and Safety Executive's Information Services database, which is used extensively within HSE, covers all industries and contains worldwide information. In addition to all the publications produced by the Health and Safety Commission and Executive, there are thousands of references to articles from prominent journals such as *Health and Safety at Work*. Legislation is referenced and the user will find the European Commission Directives, all the appropriate Acts and Statutory Instruments as well as data sheets, reports, guidance and advice, codes of practice, and translations. Over 12 000 references are added annually to the database which was started in 1977.

All these databases combine to make OSH-ROM a vital and unique resource for information concerning occupational health and safety whatever the industry. These databases together contain over 300 000 citations taken from 500 journals and 100 000 reports and publications. OSH-ROM is available from SilverPlatter Information Ltd.

OSH-CD gives the full text of all the appropriate legislation, including Acts and Statutory Instruments in the United Kingdom, and all the publications from the Health and Safety Commission and Executive. The OSH manager will find authorized and approved lists, codes of practice, guidance notes, research reports, methods for determination of hazardous substances, toxicity reviews, etc. Likewise the full text of all the journals such as *Toxic Substances Bulletin, HSC Newsletter* and *Radiation Adviser*. In addition there are abstracts of over 1400 British Standard Specifications concerned with health and safety at work.

Over 5000 documents are in OSH-CD and the numbers are increasing with every update, for example, the latest update will contain the CHIP regulations and associated documents. Searching OSH-CD is easy and quick and will surprise the searcher with the wealth of detail. A search of the latest edition for 'record keeping' will reveal 107 records in a matter of seconds. Compare the time which would be spent trying to locate this detail by physically searching all the documents.

OSH OFFSHORE, launched in May 1993, gives unlimited access to essential health and safety information specifically relevant to the offshore oil and gas industry. It contains the full text of all relevant legislation and guidance from the Health and Safety Commission and Executive, all Offshore Technology Reports – OTH and OTI series, operations notices, the two volume Cullen report on the Piper Alpha Disaster and the transcripts of the 180-day Piper Alpha inquiry. In addition, the full text of journals such as *Offshore Research Focus, HSC Newsletter* and *Toxic Substances Bulletin* are contained OSH OFFSHORE.

OSH-CD and OSH OFFSHORE are jointly produced by the Health and Safety Information Services, HMSO and SilverPlatter Information Ltd.

There are a number of other databases and CD-ROMs which are relevant to the OSH manager and will give specific information, e.g. CCINFO CD-ROM from the Canadian Centre of Occupational Health and Safety in Hamilton, Canada; Hazdata from the National Chemical Emergency Centre, Harwell, UK; CORDIS CD-ROM giving details of the various European Union research and development databases; databases from the Royal Society of Chemistry, Cambridge, UK; and Environmental Health on CD-ROM published by Context Electronic Publishers, London.

New CD-ROMs that will assist the OSH manager are in preparation and will be ready in 1994/95. Amongst these are the new Technical

Indexes Occupational Health and Safety Information Service; and HMSO and SilverPlatter's new *Fire* and *Food Safety* (with others in the pipeline). There is a constant stream of new OSH information, and by harnessing the power of the computer and the compact disc technology access to this wealth of authoritative and validated information is easy and should be available in all OSH managers' offices.

BSI STANDARDLINE

The BSI database, BSI Standardline, lists all standards and is publicly available online through a host computer system besides being available on the Perinorm CD-ROM. The BSI Standardline gives a tremendous amount of information not found in the printed catalogues, including a complete list of all the amendments, corresponding international standards, subjects, designation codes, and committee references. The user can have automatic searches carried out on a tailormade service. Contact BSI for details.

PERINORM is the world's first multinational, multilingual standards database available on compact disc. It gives you touch-of-a-button access to current information on British, French, German, Austrian, Swiss, European and international standards, as well as French and German technical regulations. It enables you to identify standards and regulations relevant to your products, check the current status of documents and keep pace with the EC's standards harmonization programme – information which can be crucial to commercial success.

It is available on annual subscription and you receive a new, updated disc every month for a year. Because you can use the directory as often and for as long as you wish without accumulating usage costs it can be very cost effective. The clear and concise instructions guide you to the information you need quickly and simply. The CD-ROM is multilingual – instructions, information and searching procedures being available in English, French or German.

The Perinorm CD-ROM can be purchased on subscription from Technical Indexes Ltd, Willoughby Rd, Bracknell, Berkshire RG12 4DW, Tel: +44 (0)1344 426311, Fax: +44 (0)1344 424971, Telex: 849207 TEKINF G. Perinorm is officially produced by BSI, DIN and AFNOR, and offers complete cross-referencing between these important European standards. Technical Indexes Ltd is the principal agent for PERINORM in the UK and also supplies BSS in microfiche and microfoil format. This service includes all amendments and revisions, with monthly updates, or it can be industry specific so that the subscriber takes only the information needed. Technical Indexes produces CD-ROMs containing full text of all British Standards.

STANDARDS INFODISK is produced by the ILI (Infonorme London

Information), Index House, Ascot, Berkshire SL5 7EU, Tel: +44 (0)1344 874343, Fax: +44 (0)1344 291194 and is a bibliographic CD-ROM containing details of over 200 000 national and international standards from more than 60 issuing authorities worldwide. All the information comes from official sources. STANDARDS INFODISK is updated every 13 weeks, has a number of unique features, including three different search modes, and is the only CD-ROM system to cover British, European, American (e.g. API, ANSI, ASME), Japanese, Australian, Canadian and international standards.

TECHNOLOGY ADVANCEMENT

Technology continues to advance rapidly, with new developments such as the worldwide delivery of high bandwidth information at high-speed transmission speeds becoming more available at ever lower costs. The use of electronic mail is also making access to information easier; even seeking guidance and advice from specialists around the world is becoming much simpler. The take-up and use of facsimile transmission of data has made a valuable contribution, again at low cost. The potential of these new information technologies is enormous. Their facilities for accessing the needed information at ever lower costs can increasingly help to reduce existing disparities in the availability of information between countries and between regions in a country. As the information delivery networks expand and further innovative applications are created using these beneficial technologies, more and more people will be reached, so that the role of information as a means of accomplishing desired changes in the workplace may be realized.

The use of electronic mail, particularly the Internet, is opening up more data sources. For the OSH information seeker this is good news – where the data is located is irrelevant; the main requirement is that the access is easy and 'seamless', gives value for money, and good easily understandable information which has been validated and is authoritative.

COST BENEFIT OF TECHNOLOGY

New technologies are also a boon to developing countries. It is well known that knowledge and information are vital to achieving improved quality of life and quality of the environment. Information technologies present one of the most cost-effective means for developing countries to keep pace with progress in the various fields of activity. Electronic technologies can substantially enhance the ability of developing countries to achieve the benefits of improved information dissemination in a cost-effective manner.

Mainframes and online systems, whilst they are by no means obsolete, are costly for many institutions. Costs such as data production and telecommunications charges are high and often prohibitive. Today's technologies, such as CD-ROM, are the best way for these countries to be informed and to come to terms with current knowledge in many areas, especially the very critical ones relating to health. The advantages that they offer for presenting large collections of information in forms that speak directly to the users, and quickly and conveniently meet their diverse needs are undeniable.

Costs of an entire workstation – personal computer, CD-ROM reader and their applications – are falling rapidly worldwide and, even in developing countries, are affordable and plentiful. The affordability of PC-based information and the local skills in information technologies, including computers, communications and information sciences, make the new technologies a desirable alternative for developing countries. They provide these countries with an opportunity to conduct activities using vital information on the same level as the developed world.

CONCLUSIONS

Information is therefore vital in today's society; it is needed in every walk of life but none more so than in the occupational safety and health field. For the OSH manager this will mean up-to-date knowledge of the legislation including the European Union directives, and the various interpretations, guidance, advice, research results, materials safety data sheets, standard specifications, details of organizations concerned with health and safety, training requirements, and awareness of films and videos which may assist in training.

In today's technology based OSH information world there is a need to be constantly asking if the data held is current. The information seeker and provider will need to keep all networks (both technical and personal) open to ensure that the information is up to date, authoritative and validated. Knowledge of a solution to a workplace hazard or potential hazard is essential if a healthy and safe working environment is to be achieved for all workers wherever they are located in the world.

REFERENCES

Cherrie, J. and McGovern, B. (1993) *A Selected Annotated Booklist for Occupational Hygienists.* Institute of Occupational Medicine, 8 Roxburgh Place, Edinburgh EH8 9SU, UK. Tel: +44 (0)131 6675131, Fax: +44 (0)131 6670136.

Pantry, Sheila (1992) *Health and Safety: a guide to sources of information.* CPI, 52 High Street, St Martin's, Stamford, Lincolnshire, UK. Tel: +44 (0)1780 57300, Fax: +44 (0)1780 54333.

FURTHER READING

EUROPEAN UNION LIST OF DIRECTIVES, RECOMMENDATIONS, PROPOSALS ETC. (CURRENT APRIL 1994)

The abbreviation OJ stands for *Official Journal of the European Union*. Available in universities and public libraries and also in European Documentation Centres throughout Europe (including the UK).

Recommendation of the Commission 2188/62 and 66/462/EEC to the Member States concerning the adoption of a European schedule of occupational diseases (OJ No 81 of 31.08.1962 and No 147 of 09.08.1966)

Recommendation of the Commission 66/464/EEC of 27.07.1966 concerning the medical surveillance of workers exposed to particular hazards (OJ No 151 of 17.08.1966)

Council Directive 77/576/EEC of 25 July 1977 on the approximation of the laws, regulations and administrative provisions of the Member States relating to the provision of safety signs at places of work (OJ No L 183 of 19.07.1977, p. 11)

Council Directive 78/610/EEC of 29 June 1978 on the approximation of the laws, regulations and administrative provisions of the Member States on the protection of the health of workers exposed to vinyl chloride monomer (OJ No L 197 of 22.07.78, p. 12)

Council Directive 80/1107/EEC of 27 November 1980 on the protection of workers from the risks related to exposure to chemical, physical and biological agents at work (OJ No L 327 of 03.12.1980, p. 8)

Council Directive 82/605/EEC of 28 July 1982 on the protection of workers from the risks related to exposure to metallic lead and its ionic compounds at work (OJ No L 247 of 23.08.1982, p. 12)

Council Directive 82/501/EEC of 24 June 1982 on the major accident hazards of certain industrial activities (OJ No L 230 of 05.08.1982, p. 1)

Council Directive 83/477/EEC of 19 September 1983 on the protection of workers from the risks related to exposure to asbestos at work (OJ No L 263 of 24.09.1983, p. 25)

Council Directive 86/188/EEC of 12 May 1986 on the protection of workers from the risks related to exposure to noise at work (OJ No L 137 of 24.05.1986, p. 28)

Council Directive 88/364/EEC of 9 April 1988 on the protection of workers by the proscription of specified agents and/or work activities (OJ No L 179 of 09.07.1988, p. 44)

Council Directive 88/642/EEC of 16 December 1988 amending Directive

80/1107/EEC on the protection of workers from the risks related to exposure to chemical, physical and biological agents at work (OJ No L 356 of 24.12.1988, p. 74)

Council Resolution of 21 December 1987 on safety, hygiene and health at work (OJ No C 28 of 03.02.1988, p. 1)

Commission Communication on its programme concerning safety, hygiene and health at work (OJ No C 28 of 03.02.1988, p. 3)

Council Directive 89/391/EEC of 12 June 1989 on the introduction of measures to encourage improvements in the safety and health of workers at work (OJ No L 183 of 29.06.1989, p. 1)

Council Directive 89/654/EEC of 30 November 1989 concerning the minimum safety and health requirements for the workplace (first individual directive within the meaning of Article 16(1) of Directive 89/391/EEC) (OJ No L 393 of 30.12.1989, p. 1)

Council Directive 89/655/EEC of 30 November 1989 concerning the minimum safety and health requirements for the use of work equipment by workers at work (second individual directive within the meaning of Article 16(1) of Directive 89/391/EEC) (OJ No L 393 of 30.12.1989, p. 13)

Council Directive 89/656/EEC of 30 November 1989 on the minimum health and safety requirements for the use by workers of personal protective equipment at the workplace (third individual directive within the meaning of Article 16(1) of Directive 89/391/EEC) (OJ No L 393 of 30.12.1989, p. 18)

Recommendation of the Commission of 22 May 1990 concerning the adoption of a European schedule of occupational diseases (OJ No L 160 of 26.06.1990, p. 39)

Council Directive 90/269/EEC of 29 May 1990 on the minimum health and safety requirements for the manual handling of loads where there is a risk particularly of back injury to workers (fourth individual directive within the meaning of Article 16(1) of Directive 89/391/EEC) (OJ No L 156 of 21.06.1990, p. 9)

Council Directive 90/270/EEC of 29 May 1990 on the minimum safety and health requirements for work with display screen equipment (fifth individual directive within the meaning of Article 16(1) of Directive 89/391/EEC) (OJ No L 156 of 21.06.1990, p. 14)

Council Directive 90/394/EEC of 28 June 1990 on the protection of workers from the risks related to exposure to carcinogens at work (OJ No L 196 of 26.07.1990, p. 1)

Council Directive 90/679/EEC on the protection of workers from the risks related to exposure to biological agents at work (OJ No L 374 of 31.12.1990, p. 1)

Commission Directive 91/322/EEC of 29 May 1991 on establishing indicative limit values for implementing Council Directive 80/1107/EEC on the protection of workers from the risks related to exposure to chemical, physical and biological agents at work (OJ No L 177 of 05.07.1991, p. 22)

Council Directive 91/382/EEC of 25 June 1991 amending Directive 83/477/EEC on the protection of workers from the risks related to exposure to asbestos at work (second individual directive within the meaning of Article 8 of Directive 80/1107/EEC) (OJ No L 206 of 29.07.1991, p. 16)

Council Directive 92/29/EEC of 31 March 1992 on the minimum safety and health requirements for improved medical treatment on board vessels (OJ No L 113 of 30.04.1992, p. 19)

Council Directive 92/58/EEC of 24 June 1992 concerning the minimum requirements for the provision of safety and/or health signs at work (OJ No L 245 of 26.08.1992, p. 23)

Council Directive 92/57/EEC of 24 June 1992 on the implementation of minimum safety and health requirements at temporary or mobile work sites (eighth individual directive within the meaning of Article 16(1) of Directive 89/391/EEC) (OJ No L 245 of 26.08.1992, p. 6)

Council Directive 92/85/EEC of 19 October 1992 on the introduction of measures to encourage improvements in the safety and health of pregnant workers and workers who have recently given birth or are breastfeeding (tenth individual directive within the meaning of Article 16 of Directive 89/391/EEC) (OJ No L 348 of 28.11.1992, p. 1)

Council Directive 92/91/EEC of 3 November 1992 concerning the minimum requirements for improving the safety and health protection of workers in the mineral-extracting industries through drilling (eleventh individual directive within the meaning of Article 16(1) of Directive 89/391/EEC) (OJ No L 348 of 28.11.1992, p. 9)

Council Directive 92/104/EEC of 3 December 1992 on the minimum requirements for improving the safety and health protection of workers in surface and underground mineral-extracting industries (twelfth individual directive within the meaning of Article 16(1) of Directive 89/391/EEC) (OJ No L 404 of 31.12.1992, p. 10)

Council Directive 93/88/EEC of 12 October 1993 amending Directive 90/679/EEC on the protection of workers from risks related to exposure to biological agents at work (seventh individual directive within the meaning of Article 16(1) of Directive 89/391/EEC) (OJ No L 268 of 29.10.1993, p. 71)

Council Directive 93/103/EEC concerning the minimum safety and health requirements for work on board fishing vessels (thirteenth individual directive within the meaning of Article 16(1) of Directive 89/391/EEC) (OJ No L 307 of 13.12.1993, p. 1)

Proposal for a Council Regulation (EEC) establishing a European Agency for Safety and Health at Work (OJ No C 271 of 16.10.1991, p. 3)

Amended proposal for a Council Directive concerning the minimum safety and health requirements for transport activities and workplaces on means of transport (OJ No C 294 of 30.10.1993, p. 4)

Proposal for a Council Directive on the minimum safety and health requirements regarding the exposure of workers to the risks arising from physical agents (OJ No C 77 of 18.03.1993, p. 12)

Proposal for a Council Directive on the protection of the health and safety of workers from the risks related to chemical agents at work (OJ No C 165 of 16.06.1993)

Proposal for a Council Directive amending Directive 89/655/EEC on the minimum safety and health requirements for the use of work equipment by workers at work (OJ No C 104 of 12.04.1994, p. 4)

Index

Page numbers appearing in **bold** refer to figures and page numbers appearing in *italic* refer to tables.

Cox, T., on stress in the workplace 29
Credit and accumulation transfer scheme, CATS 230
Croner's, updating services in OSH legislation 255–6, 258
CTDs, *see* Cumulative trauma disorders
Cullen, M.C., on retention of first aid knowledge 199
Cumulative trauma disorders, CTDs 148, 158–61
see also Repetitive strain injuries

Dartmouth Primary Care Co-operative Information Project, Co-op Project 82
DAS, *see* Disablement Advisory Service
Data collection, *see* Record keeping
Deacon, S.P., on screening for coronary risk factors 209–10
Deafness, work related 55, 99, 205, 213
Denning, Lord Justice, on employer responsibility 48
Dental laboratory technicians, respiratory health of 222
Department of Employment, Employment Service of 70
Department of Health, and OSH information 259, 264
Department of Social Security, DSS Industrial Injuries Schemes, II 97
on medical assessment 71
Department of Trade and Industry, and OSH information 259
Depression, work related 29, 205–6
Dermatitis, *see* Skin
Developing countries, fatal accident rates in 6–8, **9**
Diabetes, in the workplace 212–3
Diamond, P.A.M., on work-related illness in the transport industry 205, 207
Diploma of Higher Education in Community Health (Occupational Health), DipHE 233, 234
Diploma in Occupational Health Nursing 37
Disability
in the work-place 72–5
Disability leave 71–2
Disability Rights Handbook, annual publication 75
Disabled Persons (Employment) Acts (1944) and (1958) 73
Disablement Advisory Service, DAS 73
Disablement Benefit 97
Disablement Resettlement Officer, DRO 73
Disabling injury frequency rate, definition of 15
Display screen equipment
quality of, and occupational health 100, 268
Display Screen Equipment Regulations 216
Diving Operations at Work Regulations (1990) 191
Diving Operations at Work Regulations (Amended) (1990) 201
Doll, R. and Peto, J., on cancer as an occupational disease 16, 103

Dorward, A.L., on perceived roles of OHNs 40–1
Driscoll, J., on evaluation in nursing 42
DRO, *see* Disablement Resettlement Officer
Drug misuse, and employment 78–80
DSS, *see* Department of Social Security
Dugdill, L. and Springett, J., on evaluation of health promotion programmes 42–3
Dust and fumes, as health hazard 22, 33, 100

EAPs, *see* Employee Assistance Programmes
Ears
damage to in the work worklace 213
protection of 151
see also Deafness, work related
Eating habits, alteration of, in preventative medicine 27, 28
ECETOC, *see* European Chemical Industry Ecology and Toxicology Centre
Ecology and the global environment, role of OHNs 231–4
Economic factors, in under-reporting of occupational illness 219
Education Act (1839) 96
Edward, F.C., on fitness for work 23
EINECS, *see* European Inventory of Existing Commercial Chemical Substances
Elderly persons, health needs of 26
EMAs, *see* Employment Medical Advisors
EMAS, *see* Employment Medical Advisory Service
Employee Assistance Programmes, EAPs 80–1
Employee disability, pre-existing, employers' responsibilities 47
Employees, involvement in health promotion programmes 40, 42–3
Employers
duties of regulations concerning manual lifting 153–4
legal liability of 45–51
liability insurance of 51–5
motivation in health awareness programmes 37
needs of, and OHNs 232, 233–4
responsibilities of 35, 174
health and safety training 150
under the Opticians Act (1989) 150
Employers Liability (Compulsory Insurance) Act (1969) 51, 52
Employment
health screening for 83
Employment assessment, and rehabilitation for work 70–1
Employment Department's Labour Force Survey, *see* Labour Force Survey, LFS
Employment Medical Advisors, EMAs 100, 190–1, 193
Employment Medical Advisory Service EMAs 97, 190, 193
and offshore rig medics 201
Employment Nursing Advisors, ENAs 190, 193
Employment Rehabilitation Service, ERS 73